IT'S NOT WHAT YOU'RE EATING IT'S WHAT'S EATING YOU

A TEENAGER'S GUIDE TO PREVENTING EATING DISORDERS —AND LOVING YOURSELF

SHARI BRADY

Skyhorse Publishing

Copyright © 2018 by Shari Brady

All rights reserved. No part of this book may be reproduced in any manner without the express written consent of the publisher, except in the case of brief excerpts in critical reviews or articles. All inquiries should be addressed to Skyhorse Publishing, 307 West 36th Street, 11th Floor, New York, NY 10018.

Skyhorse Publishing books may be purchased in bulk at special discounts for sales promotion, corporate gifts, fund-raising, or educational purposes. Special editions can also be created to specifications. For details, contact the Special Sales Department, Skyhorse Publishing, 307 West 36th Street, 11th Floor, New York, NY 10018 or info@skyhorsepublishing.com.

Skyhorse® and Skyhorse Publishing® are registered trademarks of Skyhorse Publishing, Inc.®, a Delaware corporation.

Visit our website at www.skyhorsepublishing.com.

10 9 8 7 6 5 4 3 2 1

Library of Congress Cataloging-in-Publication Data is available on file.

Cover design by Jane Sheppard
Cover photo credit: iStockphoto

Print ISBN: 978-1-5107-2262-0
Ebook ISBN: 978-1-5107-2263-7

Printed in the United States of America

For Luke and Lucy

Contents

Part 3: Your Relationships with Others

Part 4: Putting It All Together

Introduction

Our relationship with food begins at birth and never ends. How we feel about our body and eating is a direct reflection of how we feel about ourselves. Life can be difficult and completely unfair at times, and nobody is born with the knowledge of how to navigate through its many challenges. Sometimes, turning to food becomes the only way we are able to cope with life.

Within the pages of this book, you will find questions that will help you judge your relationship with your body and yourself. Some of these questions are simple, yet profound. Are you happy with yourself? Are you happy with your body? Why or why not? Are you happy with your life? Are you taking care of yourself? Would you like to eat healthier but don't know how or where to start? Do you constantly compare yourself to others and always feel they are more attractive, thinner, smarter, and better than you? Are you constantly on a diet? Are you in a perpetual cycle of going on a diet, losing weight, going off your diet, and gaining all the weight back? Do you wonder if you have an eating disorder? Do you know you have an eating disorder—but are afraid to ask for help?

All relationships take effort, and the relationship you have with yourself is no different. Understanding why you're struggling with your weight or with food is the first step in ending the vicious cycle of dieting and obsessions with your body. Think about how good it will feel to be free from thinking about what you should or should not eat all the time. And, instead of obsessing about food, you'll be spending your time working toward building a life filled with passion and substance.

The point of this book is to help you to get to know yourself inside and out and accept who you are. Each chapter contains questions to answer, quizzes, and some expressionistic therapy exercises. In addition to those exercises, I also ask you to write down your emotions and experiences. I strongly suggest finding a journal or spiral notebook for you to record your thoughts or even use as an art therapy book—whatever works for your process. Writing or creating art can be amazingly therapeutic and an awesome way to explore who you are and what you want. Perhaps this book will be the first step you take in making your life better and will enable you to realize if you need to seek out a therapist or talk to an adult for more help. Or maybe you've already been in therapy and are looking for another way to explore your inner self. Whatever the case is, I hope in some way this book will help you feel better about yourself and your life.

Before you begin this journey, be prepared to feel a little uncomfortable. Some of the questions are going to stir up thoughts and memories and emotions; however, believe it or not, feeling things is the only way to move forward in life. Fear of feeling sad or angry or hurt is completely normal. It means you're human; nobody likes to feel negative emotions. Always keep in mind that if you think something is too much to handle, do not hesitate to ask for help.

Also included within each chapter is a brief personal note about me. My hope is that by sharing my thoughts and feelings with you, you'll feel less isolated and alone in your journey. I spent junior high through my college years at war with my body and with food. I was convinced that I was the only person on the planet with these issues and constant struggles.

Finally, I promise that if you work through this book, you'll see how normal and awesome you are—and that's what will give you the strength to walk up the ladder with confidence and self-assurance. When you step away from the suffocating thoughts and patterns that pulled you into the hole, you'll be able to breathe again and walk out into the light and the life you were meant to live.

PART 1

Your Relationship with Food

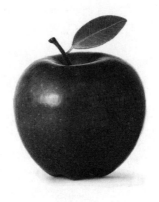

CHAPTER 1

What Is Emotional Eating?

Emotional eating refers to consumption that is triggered by something other than hunger. If you ever babysat younger brothers or sisters or small children, you'll notice that they generally do not eat for any other reason but to satisfy their own hunger. A three-year-old doesn't come home from preschool and sit down at the table and devour a whole sleeve of Oreos because they are attempting to soothe themselves after getting bullied or after they have been given a time out for purposely coloring on one of their classmates' coloring pages. If the ice cream truck comes down the street fifteen minutes after a child has just had lunch and they beg for ice cream, they will most likely only eat two bites of "Mickey Mouse on a stick" before handing the rest of the melting mess over to the nearest adult—they are no longer hungry and they don't want to eat it. Unlike adults, young children do not try to force food down because they paid six dollars for it or because they are trying to feel better about themselves after a nasty breakup with their boyfriend or girlfriend. In other words, they do not participate in emotional eating.

Emotional eating is complex. Sometimes we learn to soothe ourselves with food from our parents, who were themselves raised to turn to food as a source of comfort. But we can also teach ourselves to find solace in food in times of trouble; sometimes it is easier and less painful to eat a pint of ice cream than to sit with our emotions and truly feel them. Feeling rejected or betrayed hurts, and as humans we're wired to avoid pain. Emotional eating (or depriving yourself of food) can also be a result of feeling bad about yourself. An unhealthy relationship with yourself will cause you to have an unhealthy relationship with food, too. Food is meant to nourish our bodies and souls, but we can get into the habit of looking to food to deal with life's challenges and difficult emotions. Are you a person who eats your feelings? Or do you deprive yourself of nourishment in an attempt to deal with negative emotions? Either way, emotional eating is almost guaranteed to present health problems down the road. And depriving yourself of food, or binging and purging, will absolutely cause other issues with your body or serious health problems.

How do you know if you're an emotional eater? Ask yourself: When was the last time you truly felt hungry? If you can't think of the last time you felt hungry, that could be a sign you're eating as a response to emotions, not real hunger. Never feeling hungry could be an indication you are eating in response to your emotions.

If you believe you're an emotional eater, know that you are not alone. Emotional eating affects millions of people in this country, and it is more common than you think. A lot of people don't know how to cope with feelings like depression, isolation, or seriously low self-esteem so they attempt to self-soothe or "fix" themselves with food. Also, emotional eating is not limited to women; men suffer from emotional eating as well, regardless of culture or ethnicity.

Emotional eating can sometimes be very compulsive—in other words, an unconscious reaction. There's a sense as if you've lost control of your ability to stop eating or as if you can't control your hand from impulsively reaching for food. Have you known people who have felt so out of control that they tell you to "get these nacho-flavored tortilla chips away from me before I eat the whole bag"? This is an example of eating in response to something other than hunger and not listening to the body's cues to stop eating.

Emotional eating is an attempt to self-soothe, but unfortunately it is not going to help anyone deal with their emotions. Eating is not a healthy way to manage your moods. Of course, when you're eating something that comforts you, you might feel better in the moment. And this is what food should do—it is meant to nourish, comfort, and satisfy. But once the food is gone, the emotion will still be present. Here is the bottom line: the only solution to dealing with emotions is to sit with whatever you're feeling. Truly feel the sadness, anger, loneliness, guilt, fear, anxiety, or whatever else it is. The best way to handle your emotions is to accept them, instead of running away from these feelings or literally trying to eat them away by watching reruns of *Friends* while polishing off a pint (or two or three) of ice cream. Using food is like any other self-destructive habit. So instead of hiding behind food to avoid those feelings, run toward them. Really feel them. And yes, you will feel bad in the process, but feeling crappy is a *good* thing. It's fantastic, in fact. If you don't allow yourself to feel badly, you'll never truly appreciate feeling good about your life. Our emotions are what make us human.

Lots of studies have proven that once you allow yourself to feel these negative feelings, they *will* go away. For example, according to a study conducted by Follette and Vijay in 2009, people who suffered from PTSD (posttraumatic stress disorder) were led through mindfulness practices to assist them in recalling traumatic memories. Mindfulness enabled participants to begin healing from the trauma, as opposed to participants running away from the negative feelings surrounding the trauma. Imagine that your feelings are a chore or an unpleasant activity you don't want to do. You dread it, right? It's not fun, and it can be scary. However, once it's over, you feel better. You've done it, and there is a sense of relief. Running from feelings keeps them trapped inside of you. Confronting them and feeling them makes them less of a big deal and easier to handle. Eventually, they go away. It's that simple. If they don't and you are constantly experiencing negative feelings in certain situations that absolutely won't go away, please ask for help.

To figure out where you stand in terms of your relationship with food, answer the few questions below. Next, complete the Mood Eating Scale, which I've modified from its original version written by L. J. Jackson and R. C. Hawkins in 1980. This will help you see, in black and white, how healthy or unhealthy your relationship with food is. Once you've become aware, you can then begin to make the right changes.

> What does food mean to you?
> Do you know what it feels like to be truly hungry?
> Do you eat when you're happy, sad, bored, or lonely?
> How does not eating make you feel?
> Do you deprive yourself of food?
> How does eating or not eating make you feel about your life? Better or worse?
> Do you avoid standing up for yourself in social situations and instead eat your feelings?

Take the Quiz

Indicate how strongly you agree or disagree with each of the following statements by choosing the appropriate letter on the scale A, B, C, D, or E—A for Strongly Agree and E for Strongly Disagree.

Strongly Agree	*Somewhat Agree*	*Neutral*	*Somewhat Disagree*	*Strongly Disagree*
A	*B*	*C*	*D*	*E*

_____ 1. Eating makes me feel better when I feel overwhelmed.

_____ 2. When I am nervous, eating calms me down.

_____ 3. When I sense that people seem to dislike me, I eat.

_____ 4. Eating helps me when I'm feeling frustrated.

_____ 5. When I am extremely happy, eating makes me feel even happier.

_____ 6. If I consume a food and feel very guilty about eating it, I continue to eat more of that food or I eat other foods.

_____ 7. I eat more than usual during periods of great stress (if I break up with a boyfriend/girlfriend, during final exam week, starting college or a new job, etc.).

_____ 8. If I have an argument with someone special, eating helps soothe me.

_____ 9. I eat just to pass the time when I am bored.

_____ 10. When I feel inferior to someone, I want to eat.

_____ 11. I eat more than usual when I feel things are out of control.

_____ 12. When I'm angry with someone, eating calms me down.

_____ 13. I eat when I am disgusted with myself.

_____ 14. On days when everything seems to go wrong, I eat much more than usual.

_____ 15. I eat a lot while studying for an exam.

_____ 16. If someone makes fun of my physical appearance, I eat after it happens.

_____ 17. When I keep my feelings to myself for so long that I feel like exploding, I eat to try and feel better.

_____ 18. I eat much more than usual after failing at a task that is important to me.

_____ 19. If someone has clearly taken advantage of me, I eat to make myself feel better afterward.

_____ 20. When I am under pressure, I eat more often.

Now, give your answers a numerical score. For each A answer score 4, each B score 3, each C score 2, each D score 1, and each E score 0. The higher your score, the more likely it is that you eat in response to emotions. As you work through this book, you can take the quiz again and again to see if your responses change throughout this process of building up a good relationship with yourself.

Your score _____

Now that you've got a score, what does it mean exactly? Higher scores mean a higher tendency to turn to food for reasons other than hunger. It can also mean you might feel bad about yourself while eating. A higher score can indicate that you are more inclined to be on a diet more often. Higher scores are also linked to binge eating, which can simply be a result of being on a diet all the time as constant dieting tends to create that kind of behavior.

Emotional Eating and Dieting: Are You on a Dieting Roller Coaster?

Here's a hypothetical situation: it's Sunday night and as Stephanie crunches on an Oreo, she convinces herself that it's okay that she has just eaten twenty-four cookies because she's starting her diet tomorrow. The next day, she is proud of herself for getting through the first day of her new cabbage diet, even though she's dying to eat anything but cabbage. By Tuesday afternoon, she feels on top of the world—she's gonna have a body like a supermodel! Stephanie's stomach is flatter, she feels lighter, and she's lost a pound or two already. She's convinced this diet will be the last one she ever goes on. However, on Wednesday, the bottom falls out from under her. Cravings for real food come at her full force; she's so sick of eating cabbage for breakfast, lunch, and dinner. The cravings slowly turn into obsessions, and all she can think about after lunch are the cheeseburgers and fries she smelled in the cafeteria. Visions of food are all she can see during her boring geometry class lecture. So after school when her slim friends ask if she wants to grab a slice of pizza at the mall, where she's just been shopping and trying on clothes (that now make her feel worse about herself), she says yes. She can't handle the realities of her pathetic life any longer. While she's standing in line, she feels guilty as hell for going off her diet, and she starts making deals with herself. She tells herself that she'll just eat half a slice of pizza and count her calories when she gets home; perhaps this half slice will be a substitute for the bowl of cabbage she was supposed to eat at dinner time. But then, after she devours half the slice, she can't stop. She's starving. She hasn't eaten anything but cabbage for three days.

When Stephanie gets home, things snowball. There is a chemistry test the next day that she has totally forgotten about, and she needs to study. She hates chemistry, and about twenty minutes into studying, she's craving those potato chips she always eats when she does chemistry homework. She tries to get her mind off of the chips that are hidden away in the kitchen cabinet, but she can't. Focusing on chemistry becomes impossible. Perhaps she better eat those chips or she'll never get any studying done. More thoughts start to enter her head: she's going to fail the chemistry exam and the class, and she'll never get into the college she has wanted to attend since she was twelve. Stephanie decides to eat the chips because she had already eaten that piece of pizza and "blew" her diet; it seems crazy not to eat the chips in order to pass the chemistry test. Her future is on the line. Then, things totally fall apart. When she finishes the chips, she feels so bad about herself and is still stressed about the exam because she procrastinated. Now, she's craving ice cream. So she dives into a gallon and before she knows it, she feels like a big, fat pig. Worried about the exam and filled with guilt, she can't fall asleep.

The next day, Stephanie skips breakfast in an attempt to get back on track. She's not going to continue the crazy cabbage diet; it was stupid and worthless. She decides to skip eating all day and have a reasonable dinner. But when dinner time rolls around, she's so hungry she convinces herself she should just eat what she wants until Monday because she's no longer on a diet anyhow. And besides, she could use a break from dieting so she can search for a new diet to start on Monday. The next few days, Stephanie feels completely out of control, like a total failure. She decides she deserves to eat whatever she wants since she'll be starving by the time she gets on her next diet on Monday. But no matter what she eats, she doesn't feel satisfied. She can't seem to feel better, and she doesn't know why.

If this scenario sounds familiar at all to you, you're not alone. Personally, I know what it feels like to use food as you battle with your body, and I know it sucks. My relationship with myself and food was dysfunctional. I knew I was spiraling, but I didn't know what to do or where to go for help. I had gone from 90 pounds (I was anorexic) to 175 pounds. I had been on every diet known to man and had tried everything to lose weight, but nothing worked. I knew there had to be an answer to my problem: there were people in the world who didn't need to starve themselves or constantly diet—these people simply enjoyed eating and exercising and taking care of themselves. And so I went on a personal mission to figure out what they did and how they lived a healthy life free from dieting.

My Story

When I was thirteen, I became interested in eating healthy and spent a lot of time doing research, including visiting my local health food store, discovering unprocessed all-natural foods and supplements and gathering information from books and magazines. I had found a new passion, and by learning how to eat healthier, I felt better physically. It became a very positive step in how I felt about myself emotionally.

Then, eighth grade happened. Life started to get more complicated, and my passion turned into an obsession. Relationships with my family and friends were changing, and I didn't know why. Looking back, I now know why. These relationships were changing because *I* was changing. And while I was growing up and evolving into a teenager, I felt like I was losing who I was. I didn't know who I was becoming, and I was scared. Losing your youth can be frightening, and instead of talking to someone about this fear, I tried to hide from it. The more I tried to hide from it, the more I became focused on food. I ate as a means to feel better about my life.

But eating wasn't making me feel better about anything at all. In fact, it was making things worse. Though I was trying to figure out who I was and what I wanted in the beginning, my focus was sidetracked and I began to obsess about my looks. I started dieting, not knowing I was heading right into the eye of an eating disorder.

From the age of thirteen to twenty-three, I suffered in silence, alone. People often wonder about anorexia and how it develops. At least for me, developing anorexia didn't happen overnight. I didn't wake up one morning and decide to stop eating. It was gradual and progressive. At the time I was suffering from anorexia, it was a relatively unheard of phenomenon. Historically, anorexia has been around since the twelfth and thirteenth centuries, but the 1970s and '80s marked a time when public awareness about the disease first began.

Noticing my weight loss and worried about my refusal to eat, my mother took me to the family doctor who thought I was simply going through an adolescent phase. He sat me down and told me I was so skinny that if I didn't start eating, I would die soon. He asked me if I wanted to live or if I wanted to die, and I replied that I did not want to die. So he told me to return home and start eating. And I did. But the problem is that when you've been starving your body for a year, you cannot simply start eating and expect your body to respond in a positive way. The body responds to sudden nourishment with many physiological changes, including retaining water.

In the next three weeks following the doctor's appointment, I gained about 15 pounds, going from 90 pounds to 105 pounds. I felt huge. None of my clothes fit. Every part of my body was bigger. The worst part was, I hated myself, and the war was only beginning. I hadn't known at the time that I was attempting to deal with my negative emotions through food.

Here's a journal entry I wrote at the very beginning of my long-term struggle with food:

> This weight thing has taken over my whole mind. I'm on a starvation diet now and plan to lose 20 pounds. I weigh about 125 . . . I've been so miserable about my weight. My friends and I are fasting all weekend. Every time I want something to eat, I am going to write "I must get skinny, therefore I am not hungry." I've got to keep losing weight. I'm down to a size 5, but I've got to keep losing.

When I wrote this in my journal I was thirteen, and I had no idea that I was going to encounter a larger struggle with my body and myself.

On the next page is a photo of me, age sixteen, and a photo of me, age twenty-one. You can see that the older me is much more at peace with myself.

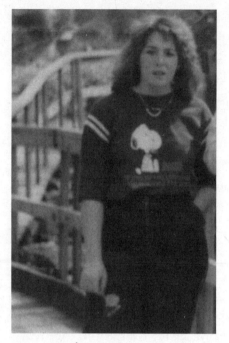

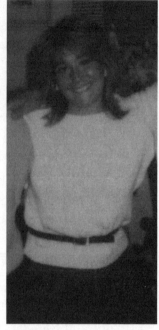

At age sixteen   At age twenty-one

Thought Journal/Food Diary

One of the ways to gather more information about your patterns of emotional eating is to keep a thought journal or food diary. They are a good way to assist people who are starting weight-loss programs. In fact, at one time in my life I worked for one of the biggest weight-loss centers in the country as a counselor, and one of the first steps in that program was to keep a journal. The journal can have various purposes, such as calorie counting or keeping track of food intake. But for the purposes of this book, the journal will not track calories. What's more critical (if you want to start making changes within you) is to keep track of what triggers your emotional eating or not eating. The journal will also help you recognize if you are feeling true hunger when you eat.

Find a small notebook you love. When you look at it, you should feel happy and positive. From the moment you get up until you go to bed, keep a record of your thoughts, emotions, and what you ate. It doesn't have to span pages; simply jot down a few words, for example: "Friends came over to hang out. Felt happy. Ate popcorn."

Be especially diligent during meal times. If you're uncomfortable writing down how you feel when you're eating with friends or family, journal before you sit down to eat or afterward. It's important to record how you feel *before* you eat, *while* you are eating, and *after* you eat to keep track of moods. Make headings at the top of the journal to help you keep things organized. Write down the time of day you're eating, where you're eating, whom you are eating with, and how much you eat. Also record how hungry you are, using a scale from 1 to 10, 1 being not hungry at all and 10 meaning you're starving. If you feel like you have an urge to eat something but your hunger is at a 2 or 3, reflect on what you're thinking and feeling at the moment. Physically writing down these thoughts can also reveal emotions you were not previously aware of. Usually, when we eat for reasons other than hunger, feelings like sadness, loneliness, anxiety, and boredom are common triggers.

Make this process easy for yourself. If it helps you, use the template on the next page, copy it onto a few pages, and staple them together to make your own journal. You can also photocopy and shrink the page to the size of a small notebook that you can easily throw into a purse, if you're constantly on the go.

Thought Journal / Food Diary

Date: _____

Time	Location/People	Amount of Food	Hunger (1–10)

Feelings/Thoughts/Emotions

_____

_____

_____

_____

_____

_____

_____

_____

Art Therapy Exercise

Find a large white sheet of paper. Draw a large circle, imagine it is a pie, and make lines (like slices) in it to illustrate different parts of your day. Delineate how your day is split-up between school, friends, part-time job, clubs or activities, family life, religious/spiritual activities, etc. For each slice of pie, think about how often food is involved and if food is the main focus. Write down a few words to describe your thoughts about how food is incorporated into the activity.

Now, look at the pie as a whole. How do you feel? Are you pretty happy with the way the pie looks, or is it kind of lopsided or empty? If the pie doesn't represent what you want your life to look like, draw a new pie to illustrate a more balanced life.

Get another sheet of paper and draw another pie circle. But this time, think about the emotions you feel throughout the day and section the pie accordingly based on how often you experience each emotion. Examples of emotions can be happy, sad, angry, worried, etc. Write down how you deal with each feeling inside the piece of pie. Next, look at the amount of pie devoted to a specific emotion. For example, is the "worry" or "anxious" section of the pie larger than the rest? Are you worried or anxious a lot? And what do you do when you're feeling that way? Do you walk the dog, watch television, or find something crunchy to munch on? Or do you lose your appetite and not eat, purposely starving yourself until the stress is over? Write all this down. These illustrations should help you see your life from a new perspective, as if you were looking at yourself from the outside. This is the first step in assessing who you are and where you're at in life—you have to know where you're at in order to know where you're going.

Finally, write down in your journal the end goals you would like to accomplish as you work through this book.

CHAPTER 2

Why Are You Eating or Not Eating?

Humans are wired to avoid any kind of emotional pain. We are also highly complicated beings. This is why therapists and psychologists spend years studying behaviors and emotions in order to help their clients sort out what's troubling them. In fact, we all begin our lives with healthy relationships with our bodies and food. To young children, eating is not complicated. However, as we grow up, the environment that surrounds us begins to influence our eating habits. Perhaps we were encouraged by others to eat when we were not hungry. Conversely (as in the case of anorexia), we may begin to deprive ourselves of food. To definitively answer the question of how someone might begin emotional eating and depriving themselves of food is almost impossible; each person is an individual with a unique biological, cultural, and emotional background. What we can do, however, is point out several reasons and possibilities that might cause someone to form an unhealthy relationship with food.

In order to move forward, it is sometimes important to look backward. In the case of trying to fix a broken relationship with food, it is helpful to examine one's childhood upbringing and how and when one's relationship with food started to get complicated.

Parenting and Upbringing

As a parent myself, I understand that parents always try to do what is best for their children. This section is not meant to blame parents for their children's faulty relationships with food. As I mentioned earlier, humans are complicated beings, and sometimes what works for one person or society or culture may not work for another. Usually, unhealthy patterns of any kind begin early and are simply a result of parents teaching their children what they think is best, depending on how they were raised.

Parents worry about their children, especially their nutrition. They worry if their children do not eat right, do not get enough vitamins, or fall sick. Personally, my parents were children of the Great Depression, as were my grandparents. Wasting food was not an option. My mother was hounded by her mother about not wasting food. She has memories of being so full and uncomfortable, only to be forced to eat more because she still had food on her plate. Luckily for us growing up, my mother was determined not to force any of her kids to finish everything on their plate. Think about the food rules at your house and all the well-intentioned attempts by your parents to influence how you eat. Take a minute and write your thoughts down in your journal. You'll most likely discover many helpful influences, as well as unhelpful ones. It's important to see both the positives and the negatives. Read through the following statements and see if you recognize anything that sounds familiar from your childhood:

- "If you finish your dinner, you can have dessert."

- "Just try one bite, it's so good."
- "Good for you! Now you're a member of the clean plate club!"
- "You can't go to school on an empty stomach. You have to eat breakfast."
- "Eat your fruit/broccoli. It's good for you."
- "Here. Open wide!"
- "You don't have to eat what I made for dinner. But the kitchen is closed after I do the dishes."
- "Do you know there are other children starving?"
- "That's fine with me. Don't eat your dinner. You'll eat it tomorrow night then."
- "You had a bad day at school? Here. Have a cookie. You'll feel better."

Parents regulate their children's diet because they want their children to be healthy. They might worry that, if unchecked, their kids will not eat enough or eat too much and gain weight. Of course, parents are also usually strict about junk and processed foods. One parent I know was so particular about what her children ate that she did not allow them to go to McDonald's. When her children eventually became teenagers and were able to eat out without their parents, a lifetime of deprivation pushed them toward making a choice for McDonald's more often. This kind of strictness, although well-intentioned, can create the opposite reaction in young adults, which is simply human nature. Parents and their children can get embroiled in these "power struggles" over food, with neither party realizing what is really at stake. If children are prevented from eating a certain food, they tend to want it even more. The forbidden fruits are always more desirable. This can lead young adults to binge on certain foods, the same way dieting forces us to feel like we need to binge.

American Food Culture

Our fast-food culture and giant processed food industries have a huge influence on what we eat. Trying to eat clean, healthy food while avoiding all processed foods is not an easy task these days. When you grow up with the same unhealthy foods being offered to you, it's very difficult to get a grip on listening to what your body needs. Humans are habitual creatures. Additionally, our lives are busier than ever. There's also peer pressure to give in to all the fast foods advertised everywhere we look. Think about how many food ads you see in a day—YouTube, television, the gas station, your inbox, Google, and Facebook. There are now even ads playing in the checkout isle. There is a real pressure by food companies to sway your taste buds in the wrong direction. In such an environment, it's pretty difficult for a bunch of kale or broccoli to compete with French fries.

It would be different if our culture didn't expose us to these unhealthy foods so early. Studies have shown that American children spend an enormous amount of time in front of the television when they are toddlers. Giving children some control over what they eat is a challenge for parents when kids are bombarded daily by only unhealthy food choices. For example, bringing a snack to school or a club or practice can be a difficult situation. You want to be popular with your peers, so showing up with apple slices or bananas can be a real dilemma. You want to be liked, so you show up with the newest Scooby-Doo cookies or Dory goldfish. Even today, as you make choices about the food you eat, think about how many of them are based on your childhood.

Your Cultural Background

Some cultures simply focus more on foods than others. My father is Italian and my mother is Hungarian; however, the Italian influence dominated since my mother grew up in a primarily Italian neighborhood. Italians are known for their food, and in my family, this was no exception. We've got the best cooks I know, and food is the cornerstone of our family gatherings. We all enjoy sitting together and talking for hours over the dinner table. Even though food is the gel that brings the family together, it does not necessarily trigger an unhealthy relationship. Sharing a meal with loved ones and participating in food rituals or traditions can be nourishing and nurturing. It is only when we start getting the idea in our heads that a food-related celebration allows us to ignore hunger cues or excuses our overeating that the trouble begins. Just because it is Thanksgiving doesn't mean there is an obligation to eat until you can't breathe or feel uncomfortable. If you feel in the mood for a second helping, go right ahead. But you should not need to feel overwhelmed with guilt or become obsessed over your choice. It's normal to overeat sometimes, especially during a special occasion.

External Eating Cues

So then, what causes us to eat or not eat? All of the reasons I've cited above can be thought of as external eating cues. When we were young, we ate when we were hungry and stopped when we were full. In the process of growing up, going to school, and becoming exposed to food marketing and the eating habits of other people, the external cues can take over your internal cues. In fact, your internal cues may soon disappear altogether. Fortunately, this basic survival instinct of eating for the sake of nourishment, though temporarily forgotten, is not gone forever. It is possible to get back to that state of being in touch with your internal cues and regaining a healthy relationship with your body.

My Story

During my long struggle with an eating disorder, there was a time when I decided to eat only on weekends. These were weekends when there would be a lot of social events involving food, and I knew I would obsess about not eating too much. I decided I needed to find a way to eat on the weekends with family and friends while still losing weight. The only solution (according to my anorexic mind-set) was to not eat at all during the week, otherwise known as fasting. From Monday through Thursday, I made sure to drink enough water and liquids that did not contain any calories. I would break the fast to eat dinner on Friday evening and continue to eat meals over the weekend. Basically, I tried to survive on water, diet soda, coffee, and tea for four days out of the week. After doing this a few times, I decided it would be a good method to control my calorie intake long term; it would also help me control my body. A few months into this kind of abuse to my body, I began to feel the effects. One of the last times I did this, I recall feeling so exhausted by Friday that I could barely walk to my classes—and forget about participating in P.E. class! My grades began to fall as well, due to the fact that my brain did not have any nourishment.

With the gift of hindsight, it is easy to see how destructive and dysfunctional my behavior was. But when you're in the midst of an eating disorder, this kind of thinking makes sense, which is why it's called a "disorder."

📝 Art Therapy Exercise

Using crayons, markers, watercolor paints, colored pencils, or even cut-out words from magazines, describe how you feel about your life right now. How do you feel about yourself? Read what you wrote in your journal over the past few days. Were you particularly happy or sad, angry or worried? Are there certain words that you use repeatedly in your journal? Use those repeated words and images as a springboard. Reflect on what you see in the words and images. What does this reveal to you? Can you see a common theme? Is there something specific you see that you want to change about your life? Do you see satisfying aspects of your life?

CHAPTER 3

Let's Talk about Eating Disorders

Before we go into detail about how to live a healthy life without depending on food, we should first define what eating disorders are and learn about the various types of eating disorders. You might be reading this book because you're tired of struggling with dieting and weight issues; you might be recovering from an eating disorder; or perhaps you'd simply like to stop obsessing about your body. The disorders listed below can be officially diagnosed by a psychotherapist, psychiatrist, or medical doctor. However, you don't have to be formally diagnosed to be suffering from the early stages of an eating disorder or from what we call "disordered eating," which refers to abnormal eating behaviors that do not fall into the strict diagnosis criteria of eating disorders. Disordered eating is much more common in our society.

What is disordered eating, exactly? When someone suffers from disordered eating, food has become the main focus of their life. Like Stephanie from Chapter 1, instead of dealing with issues and challenges, the person turns to food or restricts food intake in order to cope. Although this is not considered an eating disorder, this way of living can be exhausting and unproductive, and it takes the joy away from eating. When food becomes the focus, it can also become the enemy.

Remember: at any point while you are reading this book, if you feel any kind of concern or have major questions, please ask for help. Books like this are beneficial to readers, but books cannot replace a therapist or a doctor. If you'd like more in-depth information on any of these disorders, please visit the National Eating Disorders Association website at www.nationaleatingdisorders. org. This website also has an online eating disorder screening you can take to see if you have an issue that would require you to see a therapist or doctor for treatment.

Anorexia Nervosa

Anorexia nervosa (anorexia) is a disease whereby a person severely restricts their food intake, which leads to weight loss. To be diagnosed with anorexia, a person's weight must be significantly low, meaning less than minimally normal. Most people who suffer from this condition are dangerously underweight. For example, if a person is five-foot-five-inches tall but only weighs eighty pounds, they are significantly underweight. There are actual body mass index (BMI) numbers that sort people into mild, moderate, severe, or extreme categories of anorexia. BMI can also indicate if a person needs to lose weight. If you are interested in finding out more about your BMI, a Google search will bring up sites where you can enter your information and receive your own BMI results.

The second criterion is that a person must have an intense fear of gaining weight or becoming fat, and they will participate in activities that interfere with weight gain. These activities include obsessively counting calories, spending large amounts of time researching recipes and cooking for people but not eating anything, getting on the scale three times a day, eating only tiny amounts of food and cutting that food into tiny bites before eating, fasting for days (this means no food, just water), and/or excessive exercising. These are just some among a host of other activities someone suffering from anorexia will participate in. In my case, I was obsessed with counting calories to the point of almost driving myself crazy. I would count the number of calories in a stick of sugarless gum to be sure I wasn't consuming more than a hundred calories in a day. This is something I can tell people and laugh about now, but at the time, I was in big trouble. I'm very grateful I didn't have a severe case of anorexia, and eventually I found the strength within myself to break free from its grips. This is one mental illness that can be fatal if not treated properly. The human body must have food, water, and rest to survive. Someone who suffers from a moderate or severe case of anorexia is usually depriving themselves of at least two out of three of those key essential needs.

A third criterion necessary to diagnose anorexia is that a person must have a distorted perception of their body image. In other words, they cannot see their body as it actually is. When they look in the mirror, they see someone who is overweight or fat, though in reality they are usually so underweight their bones are sticking out from under the skin. People who suffer from anorexia also have self-esteem that is directly related to body image—how that person feels about their body is how they perceive their overall worth.

Within the category of anorexia nervosa, there are two subcategories or types: the restricting type and the binge eating or purging type. If someone suffers from the restricting type of anorexia, they will only be losing weight as a result of dieting, fasting, or excessive exercise. If they suffer from the binge eating or purging type, they lose weight primarily as a result of binge eating or purging behaviors, such as self-induced vomiting or the misuse of laxatives, diuretics, or enemas.

Bulimia Nervosa

Bulimia can also be a life-threatening eating disorder. People who are diagnosed with this disease consistently binge eat and then partake in behaviors like self-induced vomiting. A binge eating episode usually happens within a two-hour time frame, and the amount of food consumed is way more than most individuals would ever be able to consume. Feeling a strong lack of control during these binge eating episodes is also common—people who suffer from this disorder cannot control their behavior and seem to lose all sense of reality when they are consuming food in this manner. After the binge, the person will then vomit, take laxatives or diuretics, fast, or exercise excessively. The dangers related to bulimia are many. The constant binge and purge cycle wreaks havoc on the person's digestive system. Just like when a person suffers from the flu, electrolytes get imbalanced from the vomiting, which is a result of dehydration. Long-term, continuous, and frequent vomiting can also possibly rupture the esophagus.

Binge Eating Disorder

Binge eating disorder is one of the most common eating disorders in the United States, according to the National Eating Disorders Association. Approximately 1 to 5 percent of the general population suffers from binge eating disorder. It is similar to bulimia nervosa, only there is no purging or attempt to rid the body of food. Binge eating disorder can result in a person being overweight, though not necessarily. For someone to be diagnosed with binge eating disorder, they must be eating larger than normal amounts of food in very short periods of time on a regular basis. They will also be eating frequently when not hungry and experiencing severe shame associated with these eating episodes.

After reading about these eating disorders, do you wonder if you might be suffering from one? *Eat-26* is a website dedicated to helping people who might be suffering from an eating disorder. Visit www.eat-26.com and click on the box "Eating Attitudes Test with Anonymous Feedback." If you receive feedback which points to a possible eating disorder, please seek out help. Tell a parent, school counselor, therapist, or any other adult you feel you can trust. Taking the test and finding out you might be at risk is the first step to recovery, and in the end, you'll be so glad you found the courage to take action and make the right changes toward living the kind of life you want to live.

My Story

When I was thirteen, I obsessed about my body and food, which quickly turned into an eating disorder. Looking back on this difficult time in my life, I can still vividly recall having all the symptoms for anorexia. For example, I recall looking in the bathroom mirror, and even though all my ribs were all showing, I did not see myself as dangerously skinny. It's hard to explain what happens to someone who is in this state of mind, and I still wonder today how I suddenly became so unattached to reality. I remember seeing the outline of my rib bones; however, I still thought of myself as fat, convinced I needed to lose more weight. I also remember ironically feeling more satisfied with being hungry than I did feeling full. There was some kind of strange comfort in having the feeling of an empty stomach. I also recall being very defensive whenever anyone made a comment about me looking too thin. It was like I knew they were right, and if I didn't push their comments away and block out their concerns I wouldn't be able to keep myself in control of my emotions and behaviors.

The one thing that took me the longest time to recover from was the emotional battle I held within myself and refused to face. Sure, the physical act of eating again and learning to keep my body healthy was a struggle, and it took a whole lot of effort. However, the emotional baggage that put me on the road to an eating disorder in the first place was more challenging to face and deal with, especially since I didn't get the kind of professional help I needed, mostly due to the fact that there wasn't the same level of awareness and knowledge related to recovery like there is now. Quite frankly, at the time it also wasn't socially acceptable to see a therapist. This is one of the reasons I continue to encourage readers to seek out professional help if you feel you need it. We are now living in a time where asking for help is acceptable—and there's a lot of help out there.

Understand that we all go through times in our lives when we overeat, or lose our appetite when we're stressed out, or decide to eat a lot when we're not really hungry. This is perfectly normal. If you are aware of these times and food hasn't become your only source of coping, it's okay. However, if you find this scenario happening more often than you'd like, then use this book as a tool to discover new and better ways of coping with life's challenges and to find out who you truly are.

Art Therapy Exercise

Think about the times when eating brought you joy and made you feel nurtured and loved. Now, think about times when food was not used as a means to satisfy hunger and/or connect you with other people but as a means to cope with life or as a substitute for a connection with others.

Draw two dining tables below. The first table should represent memories of when food nurtured you and connected you with family and friends. When you think back on these times, you should feel peaceful and a real sense of joy.

The second table should represent the opposite: disordered eating or times when eating was not a pleasant experience. Feel free to be abstract in this exercise, and use symbols or magazine clippings for people, places, and events. Try to locate and represent the various people or events in your life that might be contributing to disordered eating.

CHAPTER 4

When Things Fall Apart— Why Do We Eat or Not Eat to Feel Better?

You now have an awareness of a few eating disorders and disordered eating. It's time to think about the process of how disordered eating occurs. Using the last art therapy exercise as a starting point, think about events, people, situations, images, and even thoughts that might occur, which can prompt the overeating or restricted eating pattern. For example, think of Stephanie who turned to food when she was feeling stressed about her homework. Are there situations in your life when you have always turned to food in order to cope?

As you go through this process of trying to change your attitude about food and your relationship with it, there is one main concept to keep in mind as you learn about yourself. Getting in touch with hunger sensations and only eating when you are truly hungry is a key concept in overcoming disordered eating.

A food journal is a great way to help you think about your relationship with food. If you have already written some journal entries, read them over and see if you notice any patterns. To help you visualize and distinguish between a healthy and unhealthy relationship with food, here is a personal example. My paternal grandmother was one hundred percent Italian and a fantastic cook. She loved to cook and bake, and she nurtured people with her gift of knowing how to make everything she made taste like heaven. Whenever I would visit her, or if we had family holidays or dinners at her house, I became aware of eating more than I normally would. This was because her food tasted so good, and sitting around the table and partaking in food was a nourishing, enjoyable activity in our family. My siblings and I would eventually expect to leave our grandmother's house with our stomachs completely full of good food, as well as a bag of goodies to take home. This is an example of simply overeating, not disordered eating. Disordered eating happens when you overeat but don't know why. Eating a whole cake or an entire bag of Oreos, while not even realizing it, is an example of disordered eating.

Use the questions below to reflect on your relationship with food and help you sort out the times when you either overeat or restrict your eating due to emotional issues, conflicts, or stressors. Write the answers in your journal.

1. When you are around certain people (friends or family), do you tend to eat more with them? If so, write their names here and think about why you overeat when you're with them. Has this become a habit simply because it is the only thing you have in common? Or do you have long talks when you get together and keep eating because you are so focused on the conversation and not aware of the food?

2. Are there people who stress you out to the point where you can't eat when you're around them? Write down who they are and why you think this is how you react to them.

3. Are there situations in which you find eating difficult because of conflict? For example, do you have family members who fight at the dinner table, causing eating to be difficult because of all the arguing and stress?

4. Sometimes you find yourself in situations or events where you might use food to cope with stress or boredom. Are there specific situations that you cannot imagine getting through without food? Try to describe them in detail.

5. Are there places that prompt you to either eat more or eat less when you are there?

6. Think about our senses that might be stimulated and make us want to eat, even if we don't realize it's happening. A good example of this is popcorn. Whenever we smell popcorn, many of us experience a very strong desire or craving to eat it; this is especially true in movie theaters. If that is the case for you, give this situation some thought. Is it the smell of the popcorn itself that compels you, or does the smell of popcorn bring you back to a time when you were younger, when your visits to movie theaters brought you happiness, excitement, and joy? Another powerful smell is that of funnel cakes at a state fair, which can trigger memories of a better time. Think about smells. Are there certain smells that trigger dysfunctional eating in you?

7. Do you notice any other situations, events, people, rituals, or places that create challenges or issues with eating (or not eating) or with food in general? Write down your thoughts in your journal.

My Story

When I was thirteen and discovered an interest in nutrition and taking care of my body—before my eating disorder really got a grip on me—I decided to attend a weight-loss camp over the summer. I was about thirty pounds overweight at the time. Since the camp was costly, I had to choose between my eighth-grade trip to Washington, DC, and weight-loss camp. I chose the latter. I was so enthusiastic about the prospect of losing weight that I began eating as healthily as I could, cutting out all junk food and candy months before my departure. By the time June came, I had already lost all my weight, but I still wanted to go to camp. This was the moment my eating disorder began. I was at a healthy weight, 125 pounds, for my size and body type, five-foot-five-inches tall. I was a size 5 or 7, but I desperately wanted skinny, pencil-thin legs like a model. *If I went to weight-loss camp,* I thought, *I could exercise, lose weight, and return home after seven weeks looking like I was ready to walk down a fashion runway.*

I only lost about seven pounds at camp since I was already within my ideal weight range of 120 to 125 pounds; plus, pencil-thin legs are just not part of my natural body shape. We worked out like crazy, and I was in the best physical health ever. I could run ten miles easily, and I looked and felt great. Most important, I learned really practical ways of eating healthy and exercising. The first thing we learned was how to become conscious of our eating behaviors. One way we were taught this was by being literally cut off from outside stimuli. We did not have cell phones or computers at that time (really). We were taken to the movies as a reward for our hard work about three times in seven weeks. Food and drink was not allowed at the movies because we were being taught to focus on the film without the distraction of food. In fact, all of our meals and snacks were eaten together in a cafeteria without any other distractions. When I left that camp, I was no longer the same in terms of my conscious eating. To this day, I cannot eat while I watch a movie. I'm glued to the screen and eating or drinking is an annoyance, much like someone talking throughout a movie.

Inspired by what I learned at camp, I created this exercise for you. I'm hoping that, like me, you'll learn how to benefit from getting more out of your movies, shows, books, etc., and you experience what it's like to be fully focused on an activity without food (or vice versa).

📝 Exercise

For the next few weeks, eat only when you are not distracted or not engaged in another activity, except for the scenario in which you are having a conversation with another person who does not stress you out. I challenge you to give up the habit of eating while watching television, videos on YouTube or Netflix, or while reading a book. Do not eat while you're studying or riding in the car; do not eat while walking or standing. Eat only while seated at a table! Try this for a few weeks, and keep a journal. The point of this exercise is to give you an opportunity to experience what it actually feels like to nourish yourself with food, focusing only on eating without any distractions.

PART 2

Your Relationship with Yourself

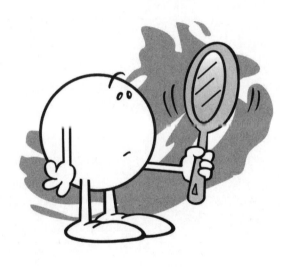

CHAPTER 5

What Are You Thinking and Feeling?

Let's go back to our hypothetical story about Stephanie from Chapter 1. If you recall, she starts her diet on a Monday, feeling positive and hopeful, then spirals into a trap of negative thinking because she can't stay on the diet. Stephanie was looking to the diet as a way to help her lose weight and, essentially, feel good about herself. She was looking outward for a solution to her unhappiness, as opposed to looking inward. Stephanie was also worried about her chemistry test, and instead of caring for herself by taking a walk, calling a friend to talk, or asking for help at school, she looked to food as a solution to calm her down and deal with her anxiety. Now, consider this. What if Stephanie tried to change the way she feels internally rather than turning outwardly to food or a diet to soothe herself?

At this point, we don't know enough about Stephanie to have an idea of how she truly feels inside. Is she depressed? Lonely? Anxious? Maybe she has a really crappy home life; perhaps her parents fight all the time or are divorced, and she misses one of them. There can be thousands of reasons why Stephanie (and the rest of us) might feel bad about life. What if Stephanie found a way to deal with her unhappiness without using food or going on a diet? What if she could gain a better awareness of what she was thinking and change her negative feelings about herself?

What we think (thoughts) determines how we feel (feelings), which influences our behavior (actions). One of the first things we should learn how to do, whenever we face challenges or wish to make positive changes in our life, is to become more familiar with our thoughts.

In the 1950s and '60s, Dr. Albert Ellis and Dr. Aaron Beck discovered that negative or unrealistic thoughts can translate into real-life problems. If a person is suffering or unhappy, the way they interpret situations usually results in inaccurate thinking. This in turn affects how they react or behave, which is usually more detrimental to the initial problem. The first step in correcting this kind of "stinking thinking" is to be fully aware of your automatic negative thoughts (the negative things you say to yourself). When you do this, you will discover thoughts that are unrealistic, inaccurate, or maybe even completely disconnected to reality.

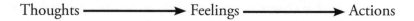

Thoughts ⟶ Feelings ⟶ Actions

Actions are what we do in response to our thoughts and feelings. For example, making the decision to eat a whole pint of Ben & Jerry's ice cream doesn't happen if it is not first triggered or stimulated by a thought, which then created a resultant feeling (like loneliness). We have the power to control our thoughts, feelings, and actions. If we are aware of this knowledge, we'll have the tools to deal more effectively with problems in our life.

The very first step in learning how to recognize your thoughts is by keeping a thought journal. Don't worry if you find that most of your thoughts appear negative. Negative thoughts are simply a part of who we are as human beings, and thinking positively doesn't come naturally to some. Understanding how negative thought patterns can be responsible for how you feel is important in learning how to deal with your life without depending on food. Thoughts create feelings, which drive our behavior, and sometimes that behavior is in the form of disordered eating.

Once you've been keeping track of your thoughts for about a week, your next step is to label them. In 1990, Dr. David Burns wrote a book entitled *The Feeling Good Handbook*, in which he uses simple words to describe negative thought patterns that lead to negative moods. Look through your journal and see if you can place one or more of these labels on your thoughts.

Step 1: Identify and Label Inaccurate Thinking

With your journal open in front of you, see if any of the thoughts you have written down fit into the ten forms of inaccurate thinking listed below. Write the appropriate label next to each thought. It is normal if your inaccurate thoughts seem to fit into several categories; most of the time they will.

All-or-nothing thinking—you only see things in black and white. If a situation falls short of perfect, you see it as a total failure. "I ate one cookie, and I blew my diet, so why not just eat the whole package and forget all about taking care of myself?"

Overgeneralization. "I ate a cookie. Now I'm never going to lose weight." Or "I always fail." Any time you use absolute words, such as *always* or *never*, to describe your behavior, you are overgeneralizing.

Mental filter. You focus on only the negatives and completely ignore the positives. Example: you have to give a presentation for history class. The whole class loves it, and many classmates compliment you afterward. The teacher gives you an A. Then one classmate tells you it sucked. Once you hear that one negative comment (which was probably a lie), you obsess about it and completely forget about the positive comments.

Discounting the positives. You insist that your accomplishments or positive qualities don't count. Example: you get a good grade on a test but tell yourself the test was so easy even a monkey could have taken it and done well. Or you insist your grade is pure luck.

Jumping to conclusions (two types):

 Mind reading: you assume you know what people are thinking or that people are already reacting negatively to you, even when there's no evidence.

 Fortune-telling: you predict things will turn out badly. Before a test you tell yourself, "I'm never going to pass it." Or before starting a new job or joining a new club you say, "No one will like me. I won't be successful. I won't enjoy myself."

Magnification or minimization. You blow problems and short-comings way out of proportion; or you shrink the importance of desirable qualities.

Inaccurate reasoning. You assume your feelings are an accurate reflection of reality, but they aren't. Example: "I feel stupid, so I must not be smart."

"Should," "must," "ought," and "have to" statements. You criticize yourself or others with *shoulds*, *shouldn'ts*, and *musts*. Look at a negative thought you've written down in your journal—is a word like *should* present? Are you constantly saying to yourself, "I should do this, I should act like this, I shouldn't have done this, I should go on a diet, I shouldn't eat this, I should eat this"? All of these phrases are very demanding. When you tell yourself that you should or shouldn't think or feel a certain way, you are essentially invalidating yourself. This can make you even more sad or anxious. Instead, replace these kinds of statements with softer phrases like "It would be nice if . . . there would be some advantages to . . . it would be preferable to . . ." These statements are much less harsh.

This technique is especially important at times in your life when events or situations happen that are out of your control, disappointing, aggravating, or painful. Life will always be testing you. It is during these times when your thoughts are most likely to veer into the negative zone. Whenever this happens, see if you can turn the unfortunate event into a learning experience or a challenge, as opposed to focusing all your energy on a negative cycle of constantly thinking, *This shouldn't have happened; I should have done this; I shouldn't have done this*. Or the infamous thought: *Why do bad things only happen to me?*

Labeling. You identify with your shortcomings. Instead of saying simply, "I made a mistake," you tell yourself, "I'm a jerk"; "I'm stupid"; or "I'm a loser."

Personalization and blame. You blame yourself for something you weren't entirely responsible for, or you blame other people and overlook the ways your own attitudes and behaviors might have contributed to the problem.

Step 2: Choose to Challenge Inaccurate Thoughts

After labeling your thoughts, learn how to manage and challenge your negative thinking. This is the next step you should take to improve your outlook. There are various ways you can do this. Since we are all unique, what works for one person won't necessarily work for another. As you read through these points, think about which method(s) will work best for you.

Examine the evidence. Now that your thoughts are placed in the categories listed above, ask yourself, "What evidence do I have that this statement is true?" For example, you might have entertained this sentiment many times: "I'll never have the body I want." Now, instead of letting that thought stay in your head unchallenged, you need to counter it. What evidence do you have that you will absolutely, positively never have the body you want? Do you have proof that this is true? If your logic is you've failed on previous diets before, that is not proof. Anyone who ever goes on a diet will "fail" some time or other; dieting is not the way to obtain a healthy body. Learning who you are, what you want, and finding out why you're not taking care of yourself is the first step you need to take to help you find the source of your pain, and then you will lose weight. In summary, you need to find solid evidence for your negative thoughts. And if you *do* have solid evidence, that's okay. Keep on reading—later in the chapter I will explain ways to deal with negative thoughts that are evidence-based, true, and painful.

The double-standard method. Look at your negative thought(s) and ask yourself, "Would I say this to my friend?" I use this question especially when I catch myself in the moment, or even when I'm simply feeling insecure. By examining your thoughts from this perspective, you'll see how hard you can be on yourself. You should treat yourself as well as you treat your friends and family. Give yourself the same kind of support you give others, and try to catch yourself in the act of being too harsh and critical.

The experimental technique. Conduct an experiment to test how valid your negative thought truly is. For example, if you experience a lot of anxiety during certain situations, such as speaking up in class, and your negative thought surrounding this is *If I speak up in class, I will make a fool of myself.* Conduct an experiment to see what would actually happen if you did raise your hand and participate. But be sure you're being fair to yourself and wait for a time when you are confident with the material being discussed in class.

Give your negative thoughts a score. This is particularly useful when facing anxiety. Although anxiety is a feeling, oftentimes thoughts—sometimes unconscious ones—create it. Rate your anxiety on a scale from 1 to 10, with 1 being very mild and 10 representing the worst anxiety you've ever felt. When you place a numbered value on your anxiety, you begin the process of accepting it. This tends to minimize its impact on you. Next, try to uncover the initial thought that provoked the anxiety, and evaluate the thought on a scale from 1 to 10 to determine its accuracy; check and see if there is any evidence to support it.

Take a survey. Ask other people if they have the same kind of negative thoughts you have. For example, if you experience negative thought patterns surrounding public speaking, ask someone else if they experience similar thoughts. You might find that your thoughts are common among the rest of your peers, which will make you feel less alone and help to minimize the negativity.

Go to the root definition of your negative thought, and then challenge it. As you journal and describe your negative thoughts in words, look up the definition of the words and challenge their meanings based on how they apply to you. Sometimes, seeing the actual definition of a word will allow you to step back and realize how harsh you are being, and it can help prevent that thought from ever returning to your mind.

Use different language. This relates to the previous point. Instead of using harsh language to express your thoughts, catch yourself and replace them with milder language. For example, instead of saying "I'm so stupid," change the words around in your head and say, "That wasn't the greatest thing I've ever done. Next time, I'll do better."

Change the thought into an opportunity to solve a problem. Instead of simply beating yourself up about something, listen harder to that negative thought and go beyond it. Focus on solving the problem. Think about all the factors that might have contributed to the situation you're in now, make a list of them, and figure out what you can do to resolve the issue.

Cost-benefit analysis. This is one of my absolute favorites. If something is not working in your life and if you continually entertain negative thoughts about it and then partake in a destructive action, write down this thought on a sheet of paper. Next, divide the paper into two columns and list the advantages and disadvantages of continuing this destructive thought pattern and behavior. Here is an example: Your life is not what you want it to be, and you constantly think, *My life sucks; nobody likes me.* These negative thoughts lead you to actions such as watching television and eating potato chips.

Write down the advantages (benefits and rewards) and disadvantages (costs and risks) of giving yourself those negative messages. Then do the same for the two related activities. List the advantages of watching television: feeling less stress, or making you laugh. Next, list the disadvantages: lack of physical exercise or avoiding self-reflection and connecting with friends or family. Do the same analysis on a more constructive behavior, such as joining a club at school, applying for a job you think you'd enjoy, joining a gym, etc. By going through this type of analysis, you'll be able to see more clearly how your thoughts and actions are affecting your life in positive or negative ways.

In addition to the methods above, there are a few other ways to handle pesky negative thoughts. According to the book *The Happiness Trap* by Dr. Russ Harris, 80 percent of our thoughts are negative or include some sort of negative content. He explains how normal this is for humans; in fact, at one time this negative thought process was useful to our survival. It allowed us to be more in tune with danger and anticipate "bad things" before they occurred. Essentially, negative thinking helped us avoid trouble. Although Dr. Harris understands how useful negative thinking was to the survival of humans in the past, he, like Dr. Ellis, also acknowledges that many of our negative thoughts lack truth and are no longer necessary for survival. Dr. Harris suggests that we should ask ourselves key questions like, "Is this thought true? Is this thought important? Is this thought helpful?"

Another device Dr. Harris suggests we can use is to understand that a thought is just a thought. *You* are not your thoughts. For example, if your thought is, *I'm going to flunk this test*, tell yourself instead, "I'm having the thought that I'm going to flunk this test." By inserting those simple words in front of the previous thought, you'll recognize that the statement does not reflect your reality; it's simply a thought.

If you're interested in visualization methods, imagine your negative thoughts floating away. I like to use the visual of balloons. If I experience a disturbing thought that I know is not grounded in truth, I imagine it as a balloon floating up into the sky. You can also imagine placing your thought in a box and putting it away on a shelf.

Or think of regular negative thought patterns as a tabloid magazine story. Whenever the same negative thought comes up, accept it as your own "celebrity gossip," and tell yourself, "Here's the tabloid story again that just isn't true." Then, let it go.

The method of accepting our negative thoughts and then releasing them can be used when faced with anxiety-inducing or stressful situations or events. For example, you are about to give a presentation at school in front of the class, and you are having strong thoughts about messing up or making a fool of yourself. So acknowledge those thoughts. Sit with them, accept them, and then let them go. By letting go, you're relinquishing them; if you were to continue focusing on them, the thoughts would grow bigger and get more intense. However, if you simply acknowledge your inaccurate thought at the outset and accept it and then imagine yourself standing in front of the class and giving a fantastic presentation, you will move past the negative thought and be able to focus your mind in a positive direction.

Another important point to consider is to be sure to pay close attention to your thoughts during times of stress and physical weakness. If you are not feeling well physically, your thought processes are not going to be normal. When you're in bed with the flu, nothing will seem positive and your thinking patterns will not be healthy. These are times when taking care of yourself is the first priority. Nurturing yourself during times of stress, illness, and trauma is vital to your health and well-being.

Lastly, there are times when acknowledging and accepting a negative thought is necessary. Earlier, I mentioned that some things happen in life that we can't control—in such situations, negative thoughts are evidence-based and warranted. In these instances, it is critical to practice acceptance. If you lose someone you love, you will certainly have thoughts about missing them, which will create strong feelings of sadness and grief. During these times, acknowledge your thoughts and accept the feelings that will follow—know that they are normal. Acknowledgment does not mean the thought should define you. You are only human; you will have good days and bad days, and you'll feel all kinds of feelings, both positive and negative.

In summary, all these techniques aim for the same end goal: replacing destructive thought patterns with constructive ones. Once you are able to recognize and identify your thoughts, you will then be able to implement the right techniques to accept or change negative thoughts into positive ones. The good news is that the more positive thoughts there are rolling around in your head all day, the more they will create good feelings within you and you won't feel the compulsion to eat, thus helping to eliminate or break the cycle of emotional eating.

Feelings vs. Emotions—How They Are Different

The words *feeling* and *emotion* are often used interchangeably because these two terms do overlap. If you were to look up their respective definitions, you would see that both words are used to describe one another. This can cause confusion, especially when one attempts to explain the two terms as two distinct neurological events that occur in our brain. Feelings and emotions can happen so quickly that it is easy to think they occur simultaneously. I'm going to explain these two processes as simply as possible. It is important for you to understand that, at times, feelings and emotions can both be used to describe a response. Other times, the words need to be used separately and distinctly to define what is going on in our brain. Even though thoughts typically precede and influence feelings, sometimes a feeling can happen to you *before* a thought if your emotions come into play.

Emotions

Emotions are instinctive responses that occur as a direct result of a biochemical reaction in the brain. Emotions assisted our ancestors in survival by producing quick, subconscious reactions to threats and rewards. Memories reside in the "emotional" part of the brain. This is why we might develop a fear of water after nearly drowning or why we may develop a fear of authority if we experienced an overly aggressive adult who yelled at us when we were young. Conversely, being lovingly fed by our parents or caregivers gives us a positive emotional response since it ensures our survival.

If a negative or positive memory pops into your mind, you will notice a physical reaction. This is an automatic response. It is a result of external stimuli prompting your brain to recall the memory that had threatened your life or given you an opportunity to thrive.

Basic emotions are instinctual and common in all of us, even among other species. For example, when humans experience joy, we smile. When dogs experience joy, they wag their tails. The emotions are the same—however, the thoughts and actions that follow vary by species.

Feelings

Feelings can occur once the emotional response hits the conscious mind. This usually happens after a shock or threat occurs. Feelings will assist you in realizing danger by putting the threat into your consciousness so you are able to take action. Feelings can also happen before thoughts if a past emotional event hidden in your subconscious is brought into consciousness. Essentially, feelings can signal the thought process. And, as we know, we are able to control our thoughts. This is why fears and phobias can be overcome if we are able to gain control over the thought process. Throughout the rest of the chapter, we will focus on feelings.

Recognizing and Labeling Feelings

Once we've identified what we're thinking, our next step is to come to terms with our feelings. Usually, we can easily connect our thoughts to a particular feeling—for example, thoughts about loss can create feelings of sadness; thoughts about not doing the right thing create feelings of guilt; thoughts about someone treating us poorly or unfairly create feelings of anger or resentment; thoughts about being alone can create feelings of loneliness. Conversely, there will be times when we are unable to recognize what we're feeling, especially during difficult or painful experiences. Our brains are hardwired to protect us, and sometimes this means coping with overwhelming stimuli by "shutting off" our feelings or minimizing what's actually happening to us. Sometimes we go into a state of complete denial. Some of us grow up without knowing how to recognize what we're feeling, or more important, what these feelings mean to us. People who struggle with feelings of depression and emptiness most of the time are likely to only feel sadness and despair. There are those who have achieved all kinds of great successes in their life but who still can't figure out why they feel as if they have a hole in their heart. In other words, their external, physical world appears to be fulfilled and whole, but their internal world lacks substance. And for some of us, this results in turning to food in an attempt to fill that emotional emptiness.

How do you know if you have a good sense of what you're feeling most of the time? Ask yourself the following questions:

- Are you unable to identify what you're feeling throughout the day?
- Are there times when you feel "bad" but can't express the reasons why?
- Are there times when you simply don't know what you're feeling at all?
- Are there times when you feel nothing, as if you're numb?
- Is this the first time you've ever thought about how you feel?
- When your friends or family ask you what's wrong, do you say, "I don't know?"

If you answered *yes* to most of these questions, you probably find it challenging to be completely in tune with your feelings. But don't worry. You *can* learn how to recognize and label your feelings. The ability to identify them and truly experience your feelings is vital if we intend to manage our life without turning to food.

But what happens when we are completely unaware of our feelings? See if you recognize any of the symptoms on this list:

- Physical symptoms, such as stomachaches, headaches, backaches

- Feeling depressed
- Sleeping too much or not being able to fall asleep or stay asleep
- Inability to focus or concentrate at school
- Lack of interest in socializing with anyone
- Lack of energy
- Inability to control anger outbursts
- Experiencing anxiety/panic attacks
- Feeling that your relationships are not very meaningful to you; feeling disconnected with your friends
- You question the purpose of living

The list above may also describe someone who is suffering from depression. In the next few chapters, I will explain how depression and other issues can manifest themselves in ineffective coping strategies such as overeating or eating disorders. But for now, let's dive deeper into how our brain operates to discover if our eating or lack of eating habits are our way of simply trying to feel *something*.

How to Recognize What You're Feeling

Recognizing what you're feeling seems to be an easy task. But if you've never really thought about this, it can be challenging for you to get into a habit of checking yourself or monitoring your feelings in the moment. The only way to know what you're feeling is to literally ask yourself, "What am I feeling?" at various times throughout the day—whenever something happens to you or whenever you suspect that you are experiencing a feeling. The best way for me to illustrate this is to go back to our friend Stephanie: the only feeling she seemed to recognize that day was guilt, which triggered her actions of dieting and binge eating. But what if she was aware of other feelings? What if we could ask Stephanie how she was feeling at the mall when she looked "terrible" in all the clothes she tried on? How was she feeling before she ate—besides just feeling "bad" about herself? Did she feel angry, sad, worthless, inadequate, unattractive, or all the above? What if she had been aware of the common feelings of anxiety for her upcoming exam? If I were able to talk to Stephanie about that day, I would ask her to describe the full spectrum of her feelings, instead of focusing narrowly on the reasons why she didn't stick with her diet. I would also ask her to think about the other days when she might have experienced the same feelings of failure and guilt over a diet.

As you move throughout your day, ask yourself: "What am I feeling?" Also ask yourself specifically: "Why am I feeling _____?" These can be difficult questions to answer, especially if you've never really thought about what you feel. For example, sadness is a feeling that can last for days or months, and it might be difficult to identify the root cause. If sadness is something you feel on a regular basis, it is important to seek out a therapist who can help you sort out the reasons why you have been feeling sad for so long. Whatever you are feeling, it is vital that you listen to what's going on *inside* your mind. Listen to your body. Listen to what your feelings are telling you, and then figure out a way to act upon them to improve your situation and, by extension, your life and the world around you. Behind every feeling there is a purpose, which is why accepting your feelings is also important, even if we don't like to feel sad or angry. They are part of being human. Accepting and acknowledging your feelings is much easier than trying to run and hide from them or deny they exist.

Once you know how to become aware of your feelings, it is important to accept them without judgement. Don't push your feelings aside or fear them. Accept them for what they are. The next step is to learn how to express those feelings without being too harsh on yourself or shaming others in the process. This is a difficult task for most, and effective communication is key when we begin to recognize, accept, and manage our feelings.

Exercises for Recognizing Your Feelings

Exercise #1

This first exercise will help you get in touch with your feelings. Next to each word in the list below, write down the last time, place, and situation you remember having that feeling.

sad _____

embarrassed _____

alone _____

lost _____

confused _____

shocked _____

tired _____

afraid _____

anxious _____

hurt _____

victimized/bullied _____

shamed _____

inadequate _____

helpless _____

indifferent _____

happy _____

open _____

joy _____

peaceful _____

loving _____

protective _____

interested _____

strong _____

positive _____

grateful _____

smart _____

caring _____

relaxed _____

attractive _____

Exercise #2

Look back on your list, and write down how these feelings manifest physically in your body. For example, when you feel seriously sad or depressed, does your chest ache? Do you feel like there's a rock in your stomach? In what parts of your body do you feel anger;

do you feel it in your head or does your heart pound? If you are feeling anxious, do you get the butterflies in your stomach? Do your hands shake?

Exercise #3

Throughout the day, ask yourself what you're feeling. Try to recognize and list simple feelings, such as happiness, sadness, or anger. Some feelings are more difficult to identify—for example, you can confuse feelings of overprotectiveness over someone with feelings of love or responsibility. At the end of the day, sit down with your journal and try to recall as many feelings as you can that you felt throughout the day. Write them down.

Exercise #4

This last exercise will help you gain more insight. Pick one feeling from the list or one that you think you feel often. Try to recognize how many times you feel that every day, and describe your experience in your journal. Keep track of your feelings, just as you did with your thoughts, to see if you experience the same feelings throughout the day or if the feeling occurs only during certain times of the day. Watch out for patterns, and keep your journaling as a record.

When you've completed these exercises, use your list of feelings as a reference whenever you need help understanding what you're feeling in a moment. Use your journal to record newly discovered feelings.

My Story

When I decided I needed to do something to get over my obsession with my body and eating, I thought about "normal" people—people who didn't seem to ever think about eating. They ate when they were hungry, they ate when they were at parties, and sometimes they would overeat during a holiday or for various other reasons. I was intrigued by "normal" people and their eating behaviors. So I decided to simply observe the people around me who were not struggling with their weight and took note of their eating habits. I also spoke to them about their relationship with food.

One of the first people I consulted with was my bestie whom I had known since first grade. I could ask her anything, and I knew her eating habits as well as I knew my own. My immediate family—my parents, my older sister, and my older brother—also did not have food issues and were a good resource. I took notice of people in restaurants and cafes. What I discovered was that people who did not struggle with weight loss or body image issues had a healthy relationship with food, meaning they used food as nourishment for their bodies and souls. Food was not used to soothe them emotionally. Once I saw this as reality, I decided to model my relationship with food in this way. I stopped dieting and stopped using food as a substitute solution for times when I felt lonely, sad, angry, or anxious. I ate small portions of everything, and if I happened to overeat for whatever reason, I would simply listen to my body afterward, which told me not to eat very much the next day. I only ate when I was hungry, and I heeded my body's cues.

My system did not work immediately. My body was such a mess from all the starving and binging and yo-yo dieting that it took me a few years to finally get back into good eating habits. And then the weight began dropping so fast, I literally had to purchase a whole new wardrobe. I will never forget the moment when I came home from college for a visit at the age of twenty-one and my older sister cried as I walked in through the door. My old pants were literally falling off of me. She knew the war was over, and so did I.

That was thirty-two years ago, and I have never looked back. I have since survived two pregnancies, gaining fifty pounds with each one. I had average-sized babies, but left the hospital with only about fifteen pounds of pregnancy weight to lose; I was in my regular jeans within a few months. During my pregnancies, I did not eat junk food or fast food, although I was known to be able to polish off a freakishly large amount of deep dish or stuffed Chicago-style pizza.

📝 Journal Exercise

As you continue to discover and label your feelings, your next step is to think about yourself in relation to other people. In other words, look at your life and put a label on all the different roles you perform. Like an actor in a play, take a step back and think about who you are with regards to others. You could be a daughter, a brother, a friend, an aunt, a cousin, a student, or a coach. Pull out your journal and write down all the roles you play on the stage of your life. Then, connect those roles to how you feel whenever you are playing them. Are there some roles you wish you didn't have? How do you manage those in your life? Are there roles you feel most comfortable in? Which ones give you the most joy, and why? The most important aspect of this exercise is for you to analyze the thoughts and emotions surrounding the many roles you play.

📝 Art Therapy Exercise

Look back on your list of feelings. Pick one, two, or three you've felt the most often lately. Using colored pencils, crayons, or even paint, express this with whatever medium you feel shows your feelings best. The most important aspect of this exercise is to allow the art to be whatever it becomes and to accept any imperfections you might see or feel as it evolves. Trust yourself and simply allow anything to happen without judgement. And remember, this is all just for you. This is not an assignment or for anyone else to see, unless you want to share it.

CHAPTER 6

Our Feelings and Eating

So far, we've worked hard to recognize our thoughts and feelings. We also know that these thoughts and feelings drive our actions. Let's return to the topic of feelings and try to categorize them appropriately in order to discover constructive ways of dealing with various feelings without depending on food. Though we experience a myriad of feelings throughout our lives, for the purposes of this chapter I'm going to focus on feelings that are most commonly related to disordered eating and eating disorders. And think of these basic feelings as an umbrella—once you learn the ways of handling them, you'll most likely be able to use the same tools to deal with other feelings as well.

Sadness and Depression

Depression, a word we hear very often these days, should not be confused with sadness. While sadness is a common human emotion, depression is a little more complex. Since depression has become such a common label in our society, I want to be sure to point out the vital differences between feelings of depression and feelings of sadness.

Sadness is a feeling in response to an event or trigger—like a thought or memory. In other words, something has to happen before a person can feel sadness. Try to recall some sad memories. When you were very young, perhaps you lost your favorite stuffed animal, which made you sad. Or perhaps you had plans to go to the beach in the middle of summer, but it rained all day. You were very disappointed, which then manifested into feelings of sadness.

Depression, on the other hand, is not sadness. It might feel similar, but it is more complex and usually happens without cause. There might have been an event that prompts feelings of sadness, but when those feelings persist and do not go away, depression might have set in. Depression physically and emotionally paralyzes people. One of the symptoms of depression is a lack of interest in doing anything besides sleeping. One of the most critical symptoms of depression is that the sufferer loses hope in everything. Feeling happiness or joy or seeing the beauty in anything is impossible. Depression can range from mild to moderate to severe. Severe depression is serious and requires the assistance of a professional therapist and psychiatrist, and it should never be left untreated.

Unlike depression, more typical feelings of sadness will eventually morph into acceptance, and eventually, you will recover. For example, you might feel initial pangs of sadness about not making the school play or getting the grade you thought you deserved on an exam. However, as time goes by you accept what happened and move on.

When humans suffer great trauma or loss in life, it is natural to experience severe sadness and grief that echoes symptoms similar to that of depression—we might feel overwhelmed with worthlessness, helplessness, and a sense of feeling sorry for ourselves. However, there is another difference between such profound feelings of sadness and clinical depression: when someone is depressed, these feelings never go away. They only see darkness in their future.

To be diagnosed with depression, a person needs to be evaluated by a therapist, psychiatrist, or sometimes a physician. A diagnosis will only be confirmed after the patient is assessed. Someone who suffers from depression must exhibit at least five of the following symptoms, which have to occur for a duration of at least two weeks. Sufferers of depression may experience varying degrees of these symptoms. If you answer *yes* to at least five of these questions, please inform a trusted adult immediately and get help.

- Are you in a depressed mood most of the day, nearly every day?
- Have you lost interest or pleasure in almost all activities, most of the day, nearly every day?
- Do you notice a significant change in your appetite or any weight changes (severe weight loss or gain)?
- Are you sleeping way too much or are you unable to sleep or stay asleep throughout the night?
- Do you feel restless often, or are you slow in your physical movements?
- Do you feel super tired and/or experience loss of energy nearly every day?
- Do you feel worthless or any unexplained excessive guilt?
- Are you unable to think, focus, concentrate, or make simple decisions nearly every day?
- Do you often think about dying or suicide?

Clinical depression can be treated, so once again, please seek out a trusted adult if you think you're suffering from depression. If you are not clinically depressed but experience feelings similar to these symptoms, you can attempt to manage them with the help of some methods I explain in this book. And if you ever feel you need more help, seek out a therapist trained in treating depression.

Return to your food journal and try to find situations where you felt sad or had feelings similar to symptoms of depression. Did these thoughts and feelings happen right before you ate? Was your eating affected by those thoughts or feelings? How accurate were the thoughts and feelings? Looking back on them, can you find any truth in what you felt? Try to see if you can substitute a more positive thought for the negative self-talk that creates these feelings.

To illustrate my point, let's go back to Stephanie. The results of Stephanie's exam come back, and her grade is a low C despite her hard work. Instead of looking at the situation through a healthy lens, Stephanie immediately begins to emotionally beat herself up. Her feelings of sadness quickly turn into depression as she tells herself she's stupid, she's never going to pass the class, and she's never going to get into her dream college, and as a result she'll never be happy. Her life is over. During the car ride home, her friend asks her what's wrong. Stephanie replies, "Nothing"; she's just tired. And then her unhealthy self-talk continues. She tells herself she's completely worthless. Stephanie doesn't realize it, but she says these negative things to herself over and over again. By the time Stephanie gets home, she's feeling so hopeless and empty inside that she marches right into the kitchen. Without thinking about what she's doing, she proceeds to open the freezer and pull out her favorite Ben & Jerry's ice cream while she thinks about how worthless she is. The pain in her heart and gut is so intense, she can hardly stand up straight. In order to make it go away, she brings the ice cream into her bedroom, plops on her bed, and begins to watch her favorite binge show. Bite by bite, Stephanie numbs the pain. She buries her despair somewhere deep inside where she can no longer feel it. But the pain returns as soon as she finishes her ice cream. Now she feels worse about herself because she didn't face her feelings and buried them instead. The most important part about this story is that Stephanie's thinking was not accurate, productive, or healthy, which led to ineffective behavior.

Now, let's see how we can change Stephanie's actions by changing her initial thoughts and reactions to her feelings. In fact, let's make things worse for Stephanie: let's give her a low D on her exam. Furthermore, she's only got a few weeks left until finals. Passing chemistry will be almost impossible. By this point, if Stephanie continues the negative self-talk of her worthlessness and hopelessness, she's not giving herself a chance to better or improve her situation, right?

Let's rewind. Stephanie sees her grade, a low D, and she feels sad about doing so poorly on her exam. She starts to worry about her ability to pass the class. However, this time, instead of spending a ton of energy beating herself up with negative thoughts and trying to hide from her sadness or bury it, let's watch Stephanie talk positively to herself as she tries to accept her sadness. As she walks down the school hallway and toward her friend's car, she still feels very sad. The difference this time is she doesn't tell herself that she's stupid or worthless; she doesn't tell herself that life is hopeless (i.e., stinking thinking). Stephanie simply accepts her sadness. She gets in the car and sits with her feelings for a minute, fully experiencing the pain in her gut and the ache in her heart. When her friend asks her what's wrong, she thinks about the reasons why she forgot to study and begins to honestly express her feelings: she didn't study enough for the exam; she wasn't prepared and almost flunked it; now she's so far behind she's not sure how she'll pass the class. Stephanie admits these thoughts to herself and tells her friend that she could have done better if she had been more proactive. Her friend sympathizes with her and shares a similar situation she was in last year. Then, Stephanie's friend offers to connect her to another friend who can tutor her in chemistry. Now, Stephanie is presented an opportunity to make a constructive change in her life. She decides to get help. She wants to take positive steps toward getting a better grade, and she will make sure she doesn't procrastinate. She decides she will do better next time, and she is determined to reach her goal. And Stephanie knows that even if she doesn't reach her goal, she will be able to accept this outcome because she had put her best effort into it.

When Stephanie gets home, she's still thinking about how disappointed she is, but she keeps telling herself that she's going to be okay; she can pass the class (constructive thinking). She's going to put a plan of action together and follow it through. Instead of heading for the kitchen, she goes up to her room, sits on her bed with her sadness, and accepts the feeling. It starts to feel less and less intense. Next, Stephanie thinks about activities that would cheer her up or make her feel good. She doesn't like to exercise, but she knows it always makes her feel better, so she puts on her workout clothes, grabs her music, and heads outside for a quick run. Stephanie also loves to make art out of recycled things, so she rewards herself with a creative walk to search for interesting things that will inspire her. This takes her mind off of her stress and makes her happy.

Anxiety

Anxiety is categorized as a feeling, emotion, and a thought. When facing a challenging situation, such as a big exam or job interview, you may feel anxious about the event and start thinking about the possibility of doing poorly on the exam or making a fool of yourself during the interview. Anxiety and panic attacks also happen if you are suppressing thoughts and feelings or recovering from trauma.

If you've ever experienced your heart racing in your chest, dizziness, an inability to catch your breath, sweating, shaking hands, an overall sense of panic and fear, or thoughts connected to a fear that you are going to fall over and die, you are probably having what is known as an anxiety or panic attack. Panic attacks happen when anxiety builds up to a point where your body literally shuts down. This is actually a normal, primal, survival response meant to protect us from danger and keep us alive. In his YouTube video "The Struggle Switch," Dr. Russ Harris explains what anxiety is and why it was useful for our survival back in the days of our ancestral cavemen. He brilliantly uses simple animation to illustrate how hormones that create feelings of anxiety helped us become aware of dangers before it was too late—if danger was present, the surge of fight-or-flight hormones made us quicker and stronger and, therefore, helped us stay alive. Conversely, panic attacks, which cause the body to shut down, also happen as a way of protecting us—if our ancestors were being chased by an animal, the severe anxiety would cause the hormones to kick in, causing muscles to weaken so the body would fall down to the ground and breathing would become extremely slow. These actions made the caveman appear to be sick or dead so the animal would lose interest in eating its prey. This kind of protective response is not necessary anymore in our contemporary world, but our modern-day anxieties can continue to build to the point of a panic attack.

It can be difficult to recognize anxiety when we don't have a specific trigger to connect it to or any way of understanding why this instinctual emotion is happening. Sometimes we feel anxiety when we're anticipating a positive outcome or when we're in a situation we fear, such as giving a presentation in class. All of these scenarios fall into the category of anxious thoughts. We saw Stephanie try to deal with her anxiety about her chemistry exam by eating ice cream and chips. The feeling of being full can at times ease the effects of anxiety and decrease the emotional response (feelings of fear and panic).

Think back to this diagram to see how our thoughts can influence our feelings.

Thoughts ⟶ Feelings ⟶ Actions

Typically, anxiety is a result of being completely immersed, some-times even trapped, in our thought process. Look back at your food journal, and see if there were times when you ate a lot as a response to anxious thoughts. Then, try and recall if there was a specific event that happened directly before or after that food entry that caused you to eat; in fact, sometimes a simple memory of a difficult time can cause you to have enough anxiety to start uncon-sciously eating. During these moments, challenge your thoughts. Ask yourself: Do my thoughts really make sense? By asking yourself questions, you help lessen the anxiety and, more important, you also allow yourself to accept that the anxiety is happening. This is the first step toward weakening its symptoms. Just as Stephanie sat with her sadness, sit with your anxiety. Trying to fight the feelings surrounding the anxiety will fuel the emotional response and your body will respond by releasing more hormones, which will continue to increase your anxiety symptoms until you faint.

Once you're able to accept the anxiety then tell yourself you're going to be okay. Focus on the reasons behind your thoughts, not the thoughts themselves. Next, think or do something else. Sometimes even something as simple as counting your steps while you're walking works. If you're at home and you suddenly catch yourself polishing off half a bag of barbecue potato chips, stop and think about your thoughts before you put the next chip in your mouth. Our actions almost always come after our thoughts and feelings, and this becomes dangerous when we are unaware of the initial thought and feeling. The main takeaway point is: learn to raise your self-awareness so you can prevent disordered eating and replace it with healthier coping mechanisms.

Practicing mindfulness is a good method to counter anxiety, disordered eating, and eating disorders. It helps you get in touch with your thoughts and feelings, and you also become more acquainted with your body's cues. You will learn to listen to your body more effectively. Our bodies actually do a pretty good job of telling us what's going on inside our minds, but we've often spent a good amount of time ignoring our body's signals. Thus, it is important to practice ways of getting back in touch with it so we can relearn how to listen to its cues. Remember how I mentioned that young children don't experience eating disorders or disordered eating? The reason is simple: when they're hungry, they eat; and when they are full, they stop. They are in tune with their body's signals and don't eat for reasons other than to satisfy their hunger. We could say that those children are mindful of their bodies. Later in the book, I will discuss mindfulness practices in more depth. For now, let's talk about mindfulness in terms of handling anxiety.

Mindfulness techniques can help you calm yourself by getting those hormones to stop surging. The brain is a powerful tool, and practicing mindfulness is a way of harnessing the power of your mind to refocus yourself and soothe troubling thoughts and feelings. It is just like the recent trend of adult coloring books, which help counter stress and anxiety. When you focus on something other than your anxiety, it will diminish. One way to do this is to pay attention to your breathing, and actively slow it down. Focus your mind on something calming and relaxing—some people imagine themselves siting on a quiet a beach or up in the mountains. Find a place in your imagination that gives you a sense of calm, and make it your own.

Anger

Anger is one of the most common reasons for disordered eating and eating disorders, because expressing anger can be uncomfortable for many of us. This is mostly due to the fact that anger is an emotion we are often told to hide because it is highly dramatic and can be connected to abusive or violent behavior. Some adults fear any expression of anger, and their kids are taught to cover it up. So, naturally, there is a huge correlation between unhealthy eating behaviors and suppressed anger. People who suffer from anorexia are notorious for not expressing their anger. Some psychologists believe that those who suffer from anorexia hold a lot of anger inside; their lack of food consumption is a means to deal with unresolved anger, which manifests itself as hurt. In fact, underneath all anger is some degree of hurt. Anger is a secondary emotion—when someone hurts us, we fly right past the hurt inside and what we feel most strongly at first is anger and rage. The more someone hurts us, the more intense our feelings of anger become.

There are two types of anger: overt and suppressed. Overt anger is expressed, and suppressed anger is buried or never expressed. Going back to your food diary, see if you experience any anger connected to your eating. Sometimes anger gets passed over for simply feeling irritated or annoyed, so watch for those feelings, too. A lot of times people are unable to feel anything *but* anger, and if this is you, just be patient. It takes a while to get in touch with what's beneath the anger.

Anger has a way of coming out of nowhere, especially if it has been building up over some time. Adolescence is a common time when fits of anger can strike without warning, and the behavior may be explosive or destructive. This is usually due to some kind of hurt or frustration that has been buried deep down and has not been allowed to surface. Anger can be stuffed down and pushed so far to a point that it may become impossible to find the underlying emotion. The first rule in dealing with anger is to accept the feeling, just as you accept your sadness or anxiety. Know that expressing anger does not mean you have to scream and yell dramatically.

In order to illustrate this point further, let's revisit Stephanie's life. This time, her parents are in the middle of a divorce battle. As soon as Stephanie hears that her parents are going to be divorced, she feels sick to her stomach, as if someone has punched her in the gut. Knowing her family is going to be torn apart feels like a huge loss to her. They will never live in the same house again; on top of that, Stephanie's brother is going away to college, which leaves her feeling like an only child. Faced with these sudden life adjustments, Stephanie feels hurt, lost, alone, scared, and sad. But instead of allowing herself to feel these extremely uncomfortable feelings and talking about her thoughts or emotions, Stephanie hides in her room and eats. She does anything and everything to avoid thinking and feeling. She watches YouTube videos and movies on Netflix, and she spends hours on social media following what the other kids are doing at school. The hole in her heart gets bigger and bigger, and as her pants start to get tighter and tighter, she feels worse about everything, especially herself. Stephanie is caught in a vicious web of self-destruction.

Six months pass, and Stephanie has gained a considerable amount of weight. She's also experiencing headaches, stomachaches, and backaches. Her mother and father can see that she's hurting, and they try to talk with her. As soon as Stephanie's mother asks her what's bothering her, Stephanie explodes. She starts screaming and yelling; she's so angry she feels as though her blood is boiling. Her hands shake, and she can barely catch her breath as she screams about how pissed off she is at her parents. However, because Stephanie has spent so much energy and time burying these unhealthy thoughts and feelings, she no longer has a clue as to why she feels so angry. All she knows is that it's her parent's fault. You can probably guess how the rest of the conversation goes from there. As Stephanie yells and blames her parents, they try to calm her down—unsuccessfully. Stephanie's pain and suffering have been going on for so long that she can't feel anything but anger toward everyone, especially herself.

In this scenario, Stephanie eats to deal with her emotions. Another possible and opposite response she could have is starving herself instead and hiding in her room, escaping in any way she can. Stephanie might also engage in unhealthy exercise behaviors—because she's so hurt by her parents' break up and feels so much anger toward them, she deals with her feelings by punishing and harming herself, and somehow these actions make her feel better. But again, the relief is short-lived. Eventually, the pain returns. Eating or not eating are virtually the same, though only *not* eating can be life-threatening.

We already know that anger is secondary to hurt. Rightfully, Stephanie is deeply hurt by her parents' divorce. But in order to not cause any more trouble in the family, Stephanie buried her thoughts and feelings. In addition, she did not talk about her pain with anyone else and did not think about how she could cope without turning to food or restricting food.

Now, what happens if Stephanie deals with her anger constructively without depriving herself of food or using food? As Stephanie's whole life is blown apart, she needs to pay close attention to her thoughts. If Stephanie quickly sits down with her journal and writes down her angry thoughts and emotions, she might notice some inaccurate thinking patterns. Some of her anger might be directed toward scenarios she is imagining, such as her brother having a great time in college without her, her parents not caring that she is alone, or the huge amount of unwarranted guilt she feels for her parents' divorce. Writing down thoughts is an amazingly simple way to observe how these thoughts, which seemed so perfectly accurate in our heads, now suddenly appear "off" once they are written on paper. And in the case where these thoughts are indeed accurate, by writing them out we are now aware of them and able to take constructive actions to help ourselves.

Next, Stephanie needs to allow herself to feel the pain related to her losses and accept what is happening to her. Stephanie can harness her hurt and communicate her sadness and anger to her parents and brother. By vocalizing her feelings to her family, she'll be able to work through them and her family can offer her emotional support. As a result, Stephanie would feel less alone.

Look over your food diary. Do you notice the times when you might have eaten more because you felt angry? Are there times when you can recall not wanting to eat in response to feelings of anger?

Boredom and Loneliness

Boredom and loneliness are the two most common reasons why people overeat. Let's return to Stephanie and her parents' divorce to illustrate how eating can become a quick fix for feelings of boredom and loneliness.

Before the divorce, Stephanie was never home alone—her brother was still in high school and her mom didn't work as late. After the divorce, however, Stephanie's mom works long hours and, at times, does not get home until after eight o'clock at night. Although her dad lives close by, he works late, too. Her brother has also just gone to college. Furthermore, after the divorce Stephanie's parents can no longer afford the house they are living in, and she moves to a new house. Now, she finds herself alone most of the time in an unfamiliar house. We can understand how Stephanie would feel sad and depressed—she's never had to be alone before, and this is an especially difficult time of adjustment for her.

Stephanie is aware that the house seems especially quiet and empty; however, it doesn't cross her mind that she is feeling lonely. All she notices is that whenever she is home alone after school, she craves something sweet. At first, she would only have a few cookies; then, a few cookies turn into a lot of cookies. Stephanie isn't aware that she is trying to solve her loneliness by filling up her stomach.

Earlier, I mentioned the importance of mindfulness and becoming aware of what our bodies are telling us. This is a good example of how our body can signal to us that we are feeling certain things—that empty feeling in the pit of Stephanie's stomach tells her she is lonely. Sure, coming home after school and taking a short break is a good idea; we all need time to decompress. But this break should be nurturing—and if the break involves a snack, the food should nourish us. You can also find an enjoyable after-school activity to do before homework if time permits—it'll help you de-stress and rejuvenate before you move into study mode.

Let's see what happens when Stephanie *is* able to cope with her loneliness in a constructive way. First, she talks to her friends who are in a similar situation, and she talks with her parents and brother about her feelings. She finds that making art helps her escape from feelings of loneliness and also gives her really positive energy when she is done with one of her creations. Stephanie joins a club or activity at school so she doesn't feel so alone; it also alleviates her boredom. She gets a part-time job after school and on weekends. These latter two actions are constructive ways for Stephanie to deal with loneliness and boredom, instead of looking to food for comfort and companionship.

Look back over your food journal and see if there were times you ate when you felt lonely. Reflect on those instances. If you feel lonely a lot and eat (or do not eat) to cope with loneliness and boredom, think about spending more time with friends and/or family. Fill your days up with activities you enjoy doing and with people who make you feel good about yourself.

My Story

When I was around twelve or thirteen, I experienced a few explosive anger outbursts over seemingly insignificant things. Looking back now at what was going on within my family at the time, the severe anger I expressed was in response to the changes occurring within my family and the extreme loneliness and isolation I was feeling but was not aware of.

I am the youngest in my family. My brother is ten years older than me, and my sister was eight years older. The big age gap between us meant a unique family dynamic, and I spent a lot of my time alone or feeling like an outsider. I quickly learned that if I wanted to hang out with the older kids, I needed to be so quiet that they would hardly notice me (my cousins, who lived nearby, were older as well). Within my own family, as well as my extended family, I was considered the "baby." Nobody meant for this to be a negative thing, and everyone in my family gave me attention and treated me with kindness and love. But there was a simple fact that couldn't be ignored: I was much younger than everyone else. Though I had siblings and cousins, I wasn't part of the group. They talked about high school stuff while I was only in grade school. They were going on dates and driving cars when I was barely old enough to ride my bike to a friend's house. I felt like an outsider.

When my older brother and sister went to college, my mother went back to work. My father always worked until nine or ten at night and was never home in the evenings. Every day after school, I spent a lot of time alone (just like Stephanie). For a while, I was able to manage the loneliness by playing my guitar until dinner time when my mother came home. It was a good and healthy coping strategy. However, the problem was I didn't take steps to face the pain of my loneliness head-on or even acknowledge that I was feeling lonely. My loneliness and isolation grew, and I became very angry with everyone in my family. I was hurt because I was lonely, but all I could feel was the anger toward my brother and sister for going to college and leaving me alone. I was angry at my parents for working and leaving me home alone so much. And I didn't know the extent of my anger toward them. All I knew was that my other friends and their families did things together, and I desperately wanted the same for me.

One Saturday, the neighborhood organized a block party. Everyone was going, including my friends and their families. My brother and sister were both visiting home from college, and I asked if they wanted to go. My sister didn't; she was hanging out with her boyfriend. My brother had plans to visit his own friends, and my parents weren't really interested either. When they all said no to the block party, I started screaming. Nobody knew what was going on, and, to be honest, I didn't, either. I remember taking my hand and sweeping it across the chess set we had on a table in our family room, sending all the pieces flying into the air. I yelled at everyone for not wanting to go the block party. I remember feeling as if nobody loved me or cared about me. And I remember feeling really tired of being so alone all the time. I missed our family, and I just wanted us to spend some time together. However, at the time I had buried my feelings of loneliness and frustration so deep that I couldn't put a name to what I was feeling. The only emotion left on the surface was my anger, and it was intense.

Eventually, enough time passed. Our family dynamic shifted a few times as I grew up, and I eventually felt us all come back together. Unfortunately, the most traumatic and hurtful change came when we lost my sister. My family was devastated. She was not only my big sister, but she had also become my best friend. My older brother and I were so overwhelmed that we didn't know what to do with our feelings when we lost her. Our first Christmas without her was only two months after her funeral, and my brother and I got into a fight in a restaurant over something stupid. We were so angry at what had happened and at ourselves; death always comes with guilt. In the middle of the argument, I excused myself from the table to take a few minutes to calm down in the ladies' room. In a fit of anger and hurt, my brother followed me in. The two of us continued our stupid argument until a woman walked in and stared at us in confusion. We realized we were not coping with our feelings constructively, and the moment we started to talk about the pain and guilt surrounding our loss, our healing began. Eventually, I was able to express my grief with the help of a therapist and work through my sadness. We all still think about her every day.

📝 Art Therapy Exercise

Write a letter you will never send to someone you are angry with. Or write a letter about an event or situation that brings up feelings of anger in you. After you write the letter, read it. As you read the letter, circle all the words that represent your feelings and make them into a list. Think about what each feeling means to you. As you read the word that represents your feelings, notice what happens in your body. For example, does your list include words like "mad," "hurt," "sad," "disappointed," or "betrayed"? Notice your body's reaction to those words. After you analyze your letter, discard it—in a dramatic or unusual way, such as disposing of it in a trash can on the street or down the trash chute in an apartment building. If you own a paper shredder, shred it to pieces . . . you get the idea.

CHAPTER 7

Body Image

How do you feel about your body? When you look in the mirror, what are the first thoughts that pop into your head? Do you see yourself as a unique, beautiful human being?

A lot of us have difficulty maintaining a healthy body image, and you may be surprised to find that most people would prefer to discuss anything besides how they feel about their body.

Historically, women and men have felt pressure to be beautiful. Fortunately, in our contemporary culture, we've acknowledged that beauty comes in a variety of shapes and sizes. Even so, according to the National Eating Disorders Association, about half a million teens struggle with an eating disorder or disordered eating. The truth is, despite some progress, our society still places a strong emphasis on being thin, and there is no way of avoiding the images we see in the media or on social media. Instead of thinking about how to achieve an unattainable super-skinny, runway-model figure, why not spend time figuring out how to feel good about the body you already live in? One thing is for certain. There is no changing our individual body type. Sure, we can lose or gain weight, but if you don't have a tiny, petite frame or, on the flipside, voluptuous curves, you're not going to be able to achieve that kind of figure.

Acceptance is the only true solution. Of course, this is a lot easier said than done—I know this, because I've been there. I spent way too many years of my life fighting my own body image, trying to be the skinny stick figure person I was never going to be. Even at my skinniest and lightest weight when I suffered from anorexia, I still had substantial legs. That's who I am. I'm not tall, and I have a definite pear shape to my body. But it wasn't easy to come to a place where I could fully accept my body, which is another reason why I wrote this book. My hope is that by the time you finish reading it, you'll feel better about yourself and all that the future holds for you.

Here are ten steps you can take to have a positive body image. Use your journal to write down your thoughts. If you're really struggling with accepting your body, please don't hesitate to ask a trusted adult for help.

1. Be grateful for your body. Think about all the amazing things it does for you every day, such as walking, running, dancing, laughing, breathing, and learning. Make a list of things your body does to help you throughout the day—from the time you wake up until you go to sleep at night.

2. Write down all the things you like about yourself that are not related to your looks or your body. On the days when you wake up feeling sad or unsure of yourself, read what you wrote. Sometimes we need to remind ourselves of our talents and gifts.

3. Look at yourself in the mirror without judgment. What would you say to a friend? Would you blurt out that she/he has fat thighs? Or a big butt? A flat chest? Or would you see your friend's body as full, shapely, and beautiful in its own way? Now, use this thought process with yourself. Write down complimentary statements about your body.

4. Take inventory of your closet. Are there clothes you have that don't complement your body type? Work with your body, not against it. Take a step back, analyze your wardrobe, and only keep the clothes that you are comfortable in and that make you feel good about yourself.

5. Think critically about the media and social media. Write about the times you notice a celebrity portraying a negative view of themselves. Are they exploiting themselves for the sake of entertainment? How does that make you feel when you see someone behaving in that way? What would you say to them?

6. This is going to sound cliché, but it must be said: true beauty comes from within. When you are feeling sad, suffering from the flu, or simply having a bad day, what does your body language reveal? How you feel inside is directly related to your outward appearance. When you feel good about yourself, you will sit up straight, walk with your head held high, and look people in the eye. Reflect on this and describe in your journal how you look when you feel good and when you're not feeling confident. Try to become more aware of what your body language says to others.

7. Be sure to nurture yourself every day. Take care of your body. Eat nourishing foods, exercise, and get plenty of rest. Find time to "unplug" and appreciate who you are.

8. Find time in your life to help others. By caring for your friends, family, and community, you can make a positive difference in their lives.

9. Remain aware of negative messages you tell yourself about your body. Replace them with positive ones.

10. Praise yourself daily for making positive changes in your life.

My Story

After recovering from anorexia, I spent many years repairing my relationship with my body and myself. I can look back and say with certainty that my negative body image started very young, and for good reason. At ten years old, I was five-foot-five-inches tall, and I had already had my first period. I was ten and fully developed, which made me extremely uncomfortable. I remember how devastated I was that I had breasts, while all my friends still had bodies like little girls. I was basically a little girl in a woman's body, and I felt like a freak. Compared to the rest of my class, I was a giant. By the time I hit middle school, some of the other girls' figures were changing, but I still felt super self-conscious. It didn't help that every other adult would mention my height and the fact that I looked so "mature."

I believe the war with my body began then. I was angry at my body for developing so quickly that it became very difficult to go to school for all kinds of reasons. I remember trying hard to hide the big secret of my body from my friends; I was terrified they would make fun of me. Instead of wearing a bra, I would flatten my chest by wearing three or four T-shirts. Unable to be honest with my friends, I felt like an outsider and an imposter, and I began to distance myself from them. I was simply too young to handle what was happening. By the time my anorexia kicked in, I felt like my mind and body were two completely separate entities. I was trying to detach myself from my body, and starving myself seemed to be the only way to punish my body for betraying me.

After going through the recovery process and discovering who I was and what I wanted, I finally got to a place where I could accept myself and my body. Almost every day, I practice gratitude for my health and well-being no matter what, because I don't take those things for granted anymore.

✏️ Art Therapy Exercise

Draw a body outline or trace a head-to-toe human silhouette from a magazine—any image you feel represents your body. Then, choose physical aspects of yourself that you like or feel positive about—your strengths. Draw these features onto the body outline and make them stand out. Think about why you have chosen them. For example, do you love your hair, and if so, why? Is it easy to style in different ways? Are you able to convey various moods or your personality with it? Explore the best parts of you, identify the reasons why, and express this in your art creation.

CHAPTER 8

How to Nurture Yourself without Food

Nurturing Activities

We often engage in interests and activities that nurture our souls. For example, taking a walk, riding a bike, or talking to a friend are good for us and can enrich our lives. However, if we don't have activities that fulfill us in this way, the act of eating can become a poor substitute to fill the missing gap.

Take a look at your journal or food diary and see if you've ever eaten because you felt bored or lonely. Note these moments—these are times when another more fulfilling or nurturing activity could make you feel better instead of eating. Basically, whenever food is used as a substitute for anything other than satisfying hunger, we should replace it with an activity that adds constructively to our life. For example, if you find yourself eating when you feel stressed out about an exam, make a list of alternative activities not involving food that will relieve your anxiety—take the dog for a walk, clean your room, or go to a yoga class. Using your journal, write down as many activities as you can think of that would be enjoyable and nurturing to you.

If you're having trouble making this list, think about anything and everything you enjoy doing, then examine the details of each activity. Do you enjoy watching certain performers on YouTube? What do they do that interests you; are they teaching their followers how to put on make-up? Think about why that person interests you—are they funny, insightful, open, and honest with their followers? What aspect of yourself do you see in them? Do you watch the History Channel a lot? Then think about making a family tree, researching your family's stories, or putting together a family recipe book. Do you watch many art shows? Explore taking an art class or simply Google how to paint or draw. Find an activity that makes you feel good while you're doing it.

Learning how to nurture yourself will take a conscious effort. Participate in activities you enjoy, and be sure you're taking care of yourself on a daily basis. This means eating healthy food, exercising, and making sure you get enough sleep and rest. Also be sure that you know what to do in difficult or stressful times. Activities that alleviate stress, such as walking, running, lifting weights, or any kind of physical activity you enjoy, is vital to your health and well-being. Knowing when you're exhausted and when you need rest is also important. For example, napping and binge-watching your favorite show might be a good alternative if you've been involved in a lot of extracurricular activities on top of school, holding down a part-time job, and only getting five hours of sleep each night. The most important key in nurturing yourself is to listen to your body. Notice when you feel physically tired or stressed or when you are so full of energy you could take on the world.

Nurturing Attitude

Let's talk about forgiveness. Having a friend hurt you or feeling the effects of a boyfriend or girlfriend's betrayal is difficult, and the whole rotten mess is painful. Parents can hurt us, as well as other close relatives. Being hurt by others is inevitable, and the key to dealing effectively with our hurt is to forgive. But sometimes this seems impossible. In some serious cases of abuse, it is unconceivable. Finally, there are a few instances when victims can heal from the scars of abuse only by accepting they will *not* forgive the abuser, by allowing themselves that option so they can move ahead in their life. But the one important thing we must all learn to do, and that is especially difficult, is to forgive ourselves. How do we do that? And how is forgiveness related to emotional eating?

Forgiveness is a difficult process that involves serious self-reflection. Most people don't understand what true forgiveness means. Forgiveness isn't about allowing someone to continue to hurt us. It also isn't about allowing someone who has offended us to be let off the hook, because people need to be accountable for their actions. Forgiving isn't about tolerating abuse or a lack of respect. Forgiveness is not playing the victim or acting like a martyr. Forgiveness is a process, not something you put on your calendar and accomplish on a Saturday afternoon. Forgiveness doesn't mean the other person(s) will change, because they may not; *we* need to change how *we* respond and feel when we're around them. Finally, forgiveness means letting go of the resentment. It's not necessarily about forgetting the hurt you were dealt but instead accepting what has happened as a small chapter in your life that you will now move forward from. You are who you are because of these past life events.

Look back on your past. Accept that you are human and that you have made some mistakes. Be compassionate. Imagine that you are filming your life story—and you're the director. Peer through the camera lens and look at yourself as a small child. How much of what happened in your past were you truly able to control? Probably not much. Children perceive the world egotistically, meaning they think the world is all about them. For example, if parents split-up, it is very common for children to think the split is because of something they did, even though there is no evidence or reality to this belief. Sometimes this unwarranted blame stays with people throughout their lives, especially if they have never taken a step back to look at the reality of the situation.

Forgiving yourself for being an emotional eater or depriver (as in anorexia) is a vital part of the process of being able to move on and affect permanent, positive changes in your life. Would you blame someone who has cancer for their disease? Do you blame other people who struggle with food, dieting, and/or eating disorders? These are questions to ask yourself as you begin the process of forgiving yourself and others, as well as the process of accepting imperfections, past mistakes, and any other bad event that happened in your life. Most importantly, it is vital to forgive yourself for wreaking havoc on your body if you've been starving yourself, yo-yo dieting, or binging. The challenge, moving forward, is learning to see yourself in a different, more positive light and appreciating all the things you have to offer this world.

Part of possessing a nurturing attitude, in addition to forgiving yourself and others, is surrounding yourself with people who are positive and supportive. This can sometimes be challenging, especially if you realize that the people you hang out with are more like your old self rather than the new person you are becoming. As humans, we constantly evolve and change during our lifetime, and the people we spend the most time with should always lift us up, not bring us down.

My Story

In my novel *Wish I Could Have Said Goodbye*, my fictional character Carmella is grieving her older sister's death. I saw her sitting in her closet with the door closed. It is a very small closet, so she has to sit on top of her shoes, but sitting there makes her feel nurtured. She could physically sit with her feelings of sadness and grief, without fear. Carmella sits in her closet a few times in the novel. And to be honest with you, once in a while when things are seriously difficult and I'm completely distraught over something, I, too, sit in my closet. This is one of my own examples of how I remain open to trying new ways of nurturing myself without using food.

Art Therapy Exercise

Grab as many magazines and/or printed materials you can find. Cut out any words that describe who you are, focusing on your positive side. Find as many as you can and glue them on the page of your journal in a way that is appealing to you. Make this a collage that will nurture and encourage you whenever you start to feel low or slip into a negative mood, such as when you are on the verge of falling back into stinking thinking. When you're done pasting the words, color or decorate it however you'd like. Place your collage in a frame on a wall or shelf where you can see it, or store it somewhere private and pull it out whenever you need it.

CHAPTER 9

Who Are You? Finding Your Sense of *Self*

Recognize Your Strengths

If someone asked you to list your twenty strengths, what would you say? In order to change your relationship with yourself and turn it into a more positive one, it is important to recognize and celebrate who you are. Dieting can sabotage self-esteem, and an eating disorder is the perfect recipe for disaster when it comes to recognizing your strengths, abilities, and talents.

Make a list of your strengths and talents. This can be difficult, but you need to come up with at least ten. They don't have to be ones like winning an Olympic gold medal, either. Start with school. What are your academic strengths? If you're not someone who gets stellar grades, think outside the classroom: What about your social life, extracurricular clubs, or anything else you participate in? If you can't find a school-related strength, what about the other areas of your life? Do you have a part-time job? How are you at home? Are you a good organizer? Do you cook? Do you help your friends with their relationship issues because you're a good listener or a problem-solver? Are you a good driver? Do you babysit? Are you able to relate to small kids? Are you skilled at handling animals? Are you very responsible? Do you dabble in music and art? If you're still struggling and believe you don't have any strengths, trust me when I say this: you *have* strengths; you just can't see them right now. Our strengths can get buried so deep that we can't find them. Consider your strengths temporarily misplaced. Keep your journal close by and a pen in hand so you can write your strengths down the minute they pop into your head.

Conversely, if you *are* aware of your skills or positive qualities, do you discount them? In other words, would you tell someone that anyone could do what you do? Do you convince yourself that your talents aren't really strengths? If so, read on. The next section might help you see yourself more clearly.

Discover Your Likes and Dislikes

Knowing what you are good at is important. It is also essential to find out what you like and what you don't like. I know this sounds pretty basic, but when food becomes the "go-to" answer in life, we can lose sight of who we are, which makes it difficult to recall what things truly bring us joy in life.

The following two sets of questions will help you sort out your likes and dislikes. When my kids were in grade school, I would use the first group as a game whenever we were standing in line or driving in the car. It helped pass the time and also assisted them in gaining a stronger sense of self. I call it the "Would You Rather . . . ?" game. Answer as best as you can, and if you don't like either choice, you can answer "neither one."

- Would you rather play a sport or be on a stage singing or acting?

- Would you rather wear a dress or pants?
- Would you rather vacation on a beach or in the mountains?
- Would you rather go to a big party or hang out at home with just a few friends?
- Would you rather see a movie or go to a play?
- Would you rather wash windows or do the laundry?
- Would you rather live in climate that has all four seasons or live someplace warm all year round?
- Would you rather have a dog, a cat, or both?
- Would you rather wear hot pink or bright yellow?
- Would you rather see a movie that's funny or dramatic?
- Would you rather see an action movie or an animated movie?
- Would you rather draw or paint a picture?
- Would you rather walk a 5K route or run it?
- Would you rather play softball or tennis?
- Would you rather study for math class or literature class?

Now answer the following questions as best as you can.

- Do you have a favorite way of expressing yourself, such as drawing or photography?
- Do you have a favorite sport you like to play?
- Do you have a favorite store where you shop for your clothes?
- Do you prefer to dress up or dress in a casual style?
- Do you know what you'd like to do after high school or college?
- Do you have fun with your friends?
- Do you feel comfortable with your friends?

- Do you feel you have a lot in common with your friends?
- What's the title of your favorite book or movie?

The list of questions can be infinite, but the point is, the more you know what you like and what you don't like, the more you know yourself. If you were able to answer most of these questions without too much thought, great—you know yourself pretty well. If answering these questions seemed fairly challenging to you, don't stress out. It just means you need to get to know yourself better, and that's okay. Use your journal to write down the things you notice you really like and do not like at the end of each day. It can be as simple as liking a certain model of car you see on the road. The more you can write about your likes and dislikes, the better. If you do this faithfully every day, your sense of self will get stronger, and it will become easier to make choices and decisions that make you happy.

My Story

When I was in high school and going through a nightmare relationship with my body and food, I felt totally fat and unattractive. I felt like I was a completely useless human being. I couldn't see my strengths at all through the clouded, distorted negative view I had created of myself. One thing I did every day, which I loved, was play the guitar and sing. It was my number one nurturing activity. However, I was a closet guitar player. No one ever heard me play except my family and my bestie, whom I knew since first grade. One night, two or three friends came over to my house. When they saw my guitar sitting in the corner of my bedroom, they were shocked. They thought that I had been lying about the fact that I played guitar. Then they saw my sheet music, my guitar picks, and my tattered music books. They urged me to play, but I said no. I was too self-conscious and scared. One of them saw a song she really liked in one of the books and convinced me to play it. As I strummed the guitar, one of my friends began smiling and swaying with the music. My other friends started singing, and so I started singing, too. They were all amazed and impressed. We sang together for the rest of the night, and I played for so long that I couldn't feel my fingertips.

A few days later at school, a guy I didn't know, who was the leader of a band, stopped me in the hallway by my locker. He said he had heard about my guitar playing and wanted to know if I would audition for his band; they really wanted a female guitar player. I was stunned. I told him no. Then, instead of backing down, he insisted I take their playlist, look it over, pick out one song, and audition for the band. I took the playlist home and stared at it. The next day, I told him I couldn't be in his band.

I still think about that missed opportunity and wonder what my life would have been like if I had the courage to take a chance on myself. I think back on that event now as a good example of how distorted and unrealistic my self-image was. I also realize that if I had known myself better at the time, I would have welcomed the opportunity to be in the band. I am a highly creative human being, and music played a major role in who I was and what made me happy. However, because I could not recognize that I was good enough, I could not make a good decision for myself.

✏️ Art Therapy Exercise

How do you see your life in the future? What are some things you want to happen next week, next month, next year, five years from now, and ten years from now? Find some old magazines, postcards, and positive notes from friends or teachers, and make a big collage full of words and pictures of your dream life—this is essentially a vision board. Focus on how you want to feel when you look at it. The purpose is to place words, images, and mementoes on the board that inspire you and make you feel positive and excited about your life. Put the board in a place where you can look at it every day so you are constantly surrounded by positivity and your dreams. The vision board will also make you conscious of what you want in your life and help you put your powerful message out into the universe.

P.S. This is your board, but I would suggest focusing on dreams that do not involve your body, food, or dieting. If you want, make a second, separate board for that topic!

CHAPTER 10

Your Life Values

Take a moment to think about your life values. Knowing your values (or what's important to you) will help you make decisions. Every day, you need to make conscious choices about what paths or roads you want to take. Some decisions are easy, and we know exactly what we want in the moment. At other times, especially when the decision is big or when either outcome carries equal benefits and drawbacks, it is very difficult to know what to do. It is common to use food as a substitute to avoid the decision-making process, especially if we've lost track of who we are and what we want.

Let's go back to our friend Stephanie. Stephanie has always been an artistic person—she enjoys art class and expressing herself creatively. However, the rest of Stephanie's family is passionate about sports. In fact, they are huge sports fans who play sports regularly—her brother went to college on a scholarship for football, her dad plays on an adult softball league, and her mother plays tennis. Before the divorce, the whole family would watch football games together on weekends, and as a family tradition, they traveled once a year to watch a college football game. Stephanie has never given any of this much thought. When she enters high school, she tries out for the swim team, the volleyball team, and the lacrosse team. Though not a good swimmer, volleyball player, or lacrosse player, Stephanie is good enough to be chosen as a member of those teams. However, she doesn't enjoy any of the practices. She is often benched or comes in last place. By the time Stephanie is a junior, her self-esteem is suffering. Stephanie uses food as a means to cope with her low self-esteem and her feelings of emptiness and worthlessness. She doesn't realize she is living a life that isn't actually hers.

When it's time to think about college, Stephanie applies to all the big state schools because they have good sports programs—she can also attend college football games every weekend. Stephanie gets accepted at these prestigious schools, and her parents are proud of her. However, she still feels like something is missing in her life. Instead of thinking about who she is and what her own values are, she uses food as a means to cope with her unhappiness and feelings of unrest. When it was time for her to declare a major, Stephanie simply choses what her parents and brother suggest—they think she should study business. Both of Stephanie's parents work for large corporations, she has never thought about doing anything else with her life. At college, Stephanie doesn't enjoy any of her classes, and weekends are not fulfilling to her either. And because Stephanie is already in the wrong world altogether, she finds it extremely difficult to connect with people. Her friendships are superficial, and she doesn't have anything in common with her roommate or any of the girls on her dorm floor. Stephanie doesn't belong. She feels empty and worthless, and the only way she can get herself out of bed is by looking forward to her morning donut. Food and eating is the *only* enjoyment Stephanie experiences in her life. Stephanie begins to gain a lot of weight, and this adds to her low self-esteem. If Stephanie doesn't start thinking about who she is and what she wants, she will never be able to make decisions that will make her happy.

How can Stephanie turn her life around? We know that she finds the most enjoyment in creativity and art, so if she begins to make decisions based on her interests, strengths, talents, and passions, it's very likely she'll be much happier. In order to truly take control of her life, Stephanie needs to become familiar with her own values. If she examines the list of values in this chapter and connects them with the rest of her passions, she'll be able to see that her life is moving in the wrong direction. It's not a wrong direction in itself; it's just the wrong direction for her.

Discovering who you are—in terms of your interests, abilities, strengths, and passions—is vital to becoming happy and living a life without needing to turn to food for comfort. Values help you stay on the right road or path, and knowing your values intimately, especially during difficult times, will help you stay motivated. Values also keep you on track or get you back on track if you lose your way. Note that values are not the same as the goals in your life. Values help you determine your goals. For example, Stephanie values creativity, and this value (when recognized and accepted) can lead her toward a possible goal of declaring an art major in college or becoming an art director.

Exercise: Find Your Values

What are values? And if you don't know what they are, how do you discover them? In your journal, create three columns:

Very Important to Me   Important to Me   Not Important to Me

I have listed eighty-three values over the next few pages. Photocopy the list, cut each value out, and place each under the appropriate category (Very Important, Important, and Not Important). Then, choose your top three to five values in each category. You should end up with a total of nine to fifteen values. You can also visit the Motivational Interviewing Network of Trainers (MINT) website, where you can print out the words in a larger font: http://www. motivationalinterviewing.org/sites/default/files/valuescardsort_0. pdf.

Look at each value carefully and really think about what it means to you. Take your time sorting them into categories. The first time I did this exercise, I was very overwhelmed. Don't stress out if your "Very Important to Me" pile is huge; this is perfectly normal! Additionally, don't feel compelled to do this quickly, as it can take a while. You might need to take a break and return to it later. Some people take a few days to complete this exercise, which can be a good approach. The idea is to continue examining your list and refining it after you give these values some serious thought. The most important part of this exercise is to meditate on what your heart and gut are telling you. Good luck!

Values List

Acceptance: to be accepted as I am
Accuracy: to be accurate in my opinions and beliefs
Achievement: to have important accomplishments
Adventure: to have new and exciting experiences
Attractiveness: to be physically attractive
Authority: to be in charge of and responsible for others
Autonomy: to be self-determined and independent
Beauty: to appreciate the beauty around me
Caring: to take care of others
Challenge: to take on difficult tasks and problems
Change: to have a life full of change and variety

Comfort: to have a pleasant and comfortable life

Commitment: to make enduring, meaningful commitments

Compassion: to feel and act out of concern for others

Contribution: to make a lasting contribution in the world

Cooperation: to work collaboratively with others

Courtesy: to be considerate and polite

Creativity: to have new and original ideas

Dependability: to be reliable and trustworthy

Duty: to carry out my duties and obligations

Ecology: to live in harmony with the environment

Excitement: to have a life full of thrills and stimulation

Faithfulness: to be loyal and true in relationships

Fame: to be known and recognized

Family: to have a happy, loving family

Fitness: to be physically fit and strong

Flexibility: to adjust to new circumstances easily

Forgiveness: to be forgiving of others

Friendship: to have close, supportive friends

Fun: to play and have fun

Generosity: to give what I have to others

Genuineness: to act in a manner that is true to who I am

God's Will: to seek and obey the will of God

Growth: to keep changing and growing

Health: to be physically well and healthy

Helpfulness: to be helpful to others

Honesty: to be honest and truthful

Hope: to maintain a positive and optimistic outlook

Humility: to be modest and unassuming

Humor: to see the humorous side of myself and the world

Independence: to be free from dependence on others

Industry: to work hard and well at my life tasks

Inner Peace: to experience personal peace

Intimacy: to share my innermost experiences with others

Justice: to promote fair and equal treatment for all

Knowledge: to learn and contribute valuable knowledge

Leisure: to take time to relax and enjoy

Loved: to be loved by those close to me

Loving: to give love to others

Mastery: to be competent in my everyday activities

Mindfulness: to live consciously and be mindful of the present
    moment

Moderation: to avoid excesses and find a middle ground

Monogamy: to have a single close, loving relationship

Non-Conformity: to question and challenge authority and
    norms

Nurturance: to take care of and nurture others

Openness: to be open to new experiences, ideas, and options

Order: to have a life that is well-ordered and organized

Passion: to have deep feelings about ideas, activities, or people

Pleasure: to feel good

Popularity: to be well-liked by many people

Power: to have control over others

Purpose: to have meaning and direction in my life

Rationality: to be guided by reason and logic

Realism: to see and act realistically and practically

Responsibility: to make and carry out responsible decisions

Risk: to take risks and chances

Romance: to have intense, exciting love in my life

Safety: to be safe and secure

Self-Acceptance: to accept myself as I am

Self-Control: to be disciplined in my own actions

Self-Esteem: to feel good about myself

Self-Knowledge: to have a deep and honest understanding of
   myself

Service: to be of service to others

Sexuality: to have an active and satisfying sex life

Simplicity: to live life simply, with minimal needs

Solitude: to have time and space where I can be apart from
   others

Spirituality: to grow and mature spiritually

Stability: to have a life that stays fairly consistent

Tolerance: to accept and respect those who differ from me

Tradition: to follow respected patterns of the past

Virtue: to live a morally pure and excellent life

Wealth: to have plenty of money

World Peace: to work to promote peace in the world

Once you have selected your values and completed your list, take
a break from the exercise and complete the art therapy exercise at
the end of this chapter.

My Story

When I was making a decision to go to college, I didn't know
what I wanted to study or what I wanted to do with my life. I
knew I wanted to help people, and I knew I loved to write. But
there were so many options, and to be honest, I wasn't supported
in my passions and what I valued by the adults around me. My
passions were new to everyone, including me. I was afraid to show
my true self, which is why my writing stayed a secret until I was
brave enough to let the world see the real me in my thirties.

   I think it is especially challenging to recognize and be true to
oneself if you grow up with interests and values that are different

from the rest of your family members. People who don't share the same passions and goals will find it difficult to understand and relate to each other. Eventually I realized the importance of living my life for me, though it took me a while to summon up the courage to accept that not everyone might agree with my decisions. There will always be someone out there who thinks I'm doing the wrong thing, and there were times when I felt very isolated, alone, and even rejected for my choices. However, in the end, I stayed true and followed my heart. I finally accepted the fact that I am the only one who can write my life story—the only one who can control my happiness. If that means having to feel alone with my hopes and dreams, so be it. In the end, I found support in the people who honestly loved and cared about me—they just needed a little time to get to know the real me.

📝 Art Therapy Exercise

This is a two-part exercise. First, write your life story in your journal. Record the events and facts from your past all the way up to the present moment. Next, I want you to write what you imagine will happen over the next few years of your life and beyond. Keep writing until you reach the point in your life where you are a grandparent or a senior. The point of this exercise is to give you an opportunity to envision your future. Try not to write with anyone else's needs or wants in mind. If you're struggling with this exercise, imagine yourself at the age of eighty or ninety, looking back on your life. What are your regrets? What are you most proud of accomplishing?

Next, on a clean, white sheet of paper, draw two roads leading in opposite directions. The first is the best road you want to travel on. Illustrate all the things you'd like to accomplish in your life—you can either draw them or paste a collage of magazine clippings. What will make you happy? Try and tie all your strengths, interests, desires, passions, and goals together, making sure your values are there, too. For example, if some of your values from the list above are adventure, authority, purpose, risk, caring, and knowledge, perhaps your best road will show you attending college and traveling to a foreign country to teach young children for a year. On the other hand, the second road should symbolize everything you *don't* want to cross on your journey. Bring all of this together into one giant work of art!

Now that you know what your life values are, we will address what you can do next in the following chapter.

CHAPTER 11

Bringing Your Values to Life

L ife is a journey and we possess the power to determine where we want to go, what we want to do, and if we will enjoy it. If we know what our values are, we are able to make choices which will lead us in the right direction. Losing sight of values and connections to others can happen when food becomes the only focus and replaces what's truly meaningful in our life (our values).

The 2006 movie *Cars* drives this message home (literally and figuratively!). The main character, Lightning McQueen, goes through his whole life so focused on the winning (his goal) that he never takes time to enjoy the journey. He also doesn't take time to appreciate the people in his life as he works toward his end goal. Because of this, our hero makes all kinds of mistakes and eventually realizes that he has not truly connected with others or himself. He discovers that he has been so preoccupied with his end goal he lost his values and his connection to others and himself along the way.

How does *Cars* relate to this book? Pursuing a single, obsessive end goal of losing weight or having an ideal body image—which doesn't exist—can result in a life much like Lightning McQueen's.

Food is a huge part of our life; it is meant to nourish us, bring us together in community, and be a source of pleasure and enjoyment. But when food becomes part of an unattainable end goal, it morphs into a source of anguish and obsession. Food becomes a chore and an enemy. We lose ourselves, our connection to others, and our values when we're consumed with such unattainable goals centered around what we eat and body image, much like Lightning McQueen, who is so focused on winning the Piston Cup Champion Auto Race that he loses sight of those things.

How then should we use our values to set the right goals that move us in the right direction? Imagine your life as a giant room, divided into four sections. Each section is devoted to an area—relationships, work/education, personal growth/health/well-being, and leisure. In the previous chapter, you chose the values you most identify with. Now, we'll examine how we can use these values to guide our life path.

I have listed these four areas below with corresponding questions. Use your journal to answer them and write down any other thoughts. As you do this, be conscious of your values and notice how they fit into each aspect of your life.

Relationships

In a later chapter, I will talk more about relationships and show you how to recognize which ones are working for you and moving you in the right direction.

- In your relationships, are you involved with people who share similar values to you?
- Are you able to freely share yourself and your values within these relationships?

- Do the people you have relationships with understand you and your values?

Work/Education

When we are of school age, we need to fulfill certain require-ments in order to reach our educational goals. Sometimes, these requirements might not fit with our personal values, and it's easy to feel conflicted and frustrated. If this is you, don't lose heart! For example, if you have to take a certain class you don't necessarily like in order to earn a degree, try to find a way to connect one of your values to the class, even if it simply means studying in a manner that allows your values to be addressed. For example, if you value order or creativity, you could utilize lists to study or write your notes in a repeating color theme. Attempt to recognize how the class is a stepping-stone that will help you achieve what you value or incorporate your values into the class by taking your own personal approach to learning. You can also find classmates who share your same values—connect with them and make getting through an unpleasant class easier and more enjoyable.

- How does your education or work fit in with your values?
- Is your education or work providing a means for you to experience your values?
- How do you feel when you are at school or work?
- Do you feel you are able to bring your values to your schooling or working experience?
- Are there people at school or work who share your value system? Who are they?

Personal Growth, Health, and Well-Being

A firm understanding of your value system will also help you discover what works best in the fields of personal growth, health, and well-being. For example, if you value being physically fit and having a moment of solitude, choose to run alone rather than join a group class at the fitness center.

- What do you currently do to take care of yourself?
- What kinds of activities align with your values, and which ones are conflicting?

Leisure

Leisure is about how you relax, unwind, or de-stress. It can overlap with the topic of self-care. Losing yourself in a book is one of the oldest and most popular leisure activities around. Binge-watching Netflix is another activity that is a completely acceptable and popular way to rest and recharge; however, note that it can become destructive when it is done in place of other responsibilities or when it is combined with binge eating (you knew that was coming!). Other types of healthy leisure activities include playing sports on a team or engaging in a creative hobby that allows for temporary escape and self-nurturing. Take the time to relax and participate in leisure activities on a regular basis.

- What kinds of activities have you thought of participating in, but have never tried?
- What kinds of relaxing activities are in line with your values?

Look back on your journal. Are you making choices in these four main areas of your life according to your values? As you proceed through this value-driven process, you might discover that you've been living your life outside of your value system. Start by identifying the area of your life that you should change right away. Change can feel overwhelming and scary, but don't worry. Be sure to approach this process one step at a time. Be patient. You'll find that many things will change automatically after one simple adjustment. You don't have to overhaul your life in a day. In the next chapter, I'll explain how to set some goals to begin this process.

Finally, remember that knowledge is power. Each day is an opportunity to make changes that will move you toward reclaiming your life on your own terms—that is, living by your values and nobody else's.

Use your journal to reflect. Which values are most important to you? If you are not living your life according to these, why not? What concrete steps can you take to begin living your life according to these values? Are there some values that you are already actively living by? How are you doing this? These questions will help you formulate a new life plan, which will in turn keep you motivated to cope with life without depending on food.

My Story

While recovering from anorexia, I became extremely frustrated when I was told to start eating and taking care of myself without any further instructions, guidance, or therapies. I had already stopped my destructive habits by then, but I didn't know what to do next. All my values were buried, and my only direction in life was grounded in being thin and beautiful. I had never given my life any thought past my body, food, and exercise. If

I wasn't exercising, I was planning my meals, and if I wasn't doing either of the two activities, I was thinking about dieting and exercising. I was constantly focused on evaluating if I had eaten too much or too little. And if that wasn't enough, most of the conversations I had with others revolved around my size, how much weight I lost (or gained), and how I had done it. There was a very real sense of success tied to my weight loss or gain and outward appearance—unknowing adults praised me for my weight loss or gain in an attempt to support my efforts to take care of my health. The problem was that when it finally came down to recovering from an eating disorder, I didn't have anything else in my life. I did not think about my values at the time and certainly not about what direction my life was heading in. Additionally, since I wasn't getting any medical guidance, I wasn't aware of my body's response to eating normally after a period of starvation. My mother took me to a doctor after I gained twenty pounds practically overnight, but he wasn't alarmed. At least I was eating and would not die of malnutrition. At that time, there was little information available about eating disorders. In fact, there were some doctors who believed eating disorders did not exist.

All of this meant that my disordered mind-set was never addressed. Even though I was eating again and on the path to recovery, I still didn't know myself and what I wanted in life. There were a number of activities in my high school that I could have participated in, but because I wasn't sure of what I wanted, everything seemed scary—plus, my self-esteem was in the toilet. I remember feeling so incredibly jealous of classmates who were clearly living a passionate life full of purpose—they were involved in things they loved and gained recognition for their hard work. One night, I had a complete meltdown in the middle of our kitchen. I stood at the counter screaming at my mother, "I just want to do something with my life!"

I still recall that feeling in the pit of my stomach. It was an ache and a desire. My mother tried to comfort me, but I couldn't hear her response. I was so caught up in my destructive thought pattern that I was unable to process her support or guidance. Essentially, I was trapping myself—shutting myself off so I remained alone and without help. This mind-set is common when someone is in the grips of an eating disorder.

I carried on with my life, struggling every single day, wondering why I was put on this earth, and isolating myself more and more. I created a life that looked and felt completely opposite of what I wanted. I knew there were other people out there living life according to their hopes, dreams, and goals every day—and then there was me. I felt like I was on the sidelines. I was a constant spectator.

What I didn't know—because I didn't get help and there wasn't much information available at the time about healing from an eating disorder or low self-esteem—was that this type of thinking and these types of feelings wouldn't magically go away without a plan. A plan of action starts when a person becomes highly aware of their own individual values. If I had known more about my values, I would have been involved with music, art, theatre, and other creative outlets in school. Although I played my guitar every day for hours on end (which acted as a very strong therapeutic modality for me and kept me stable), I also wanted desperately to write for the school newspaper, but I felt too insecure to tell anyone. Instead, I wrote in my journal and wrote letters to my siblings and cousins who were away at college (there weren't emails or cell phones at the time). Today, I understand why I had kept my interests hidden, especially writing. Any kind of self-expression requires the courage to be vulnerable. Expressing oneself to others means revealing yourself in a very genuine way. Without having recovered properly from my eating disorder, my sense of self was too weak and fragile. I hid myself from the entire world, except for my older sister, to whom I wrote a lot of letters. She knew I kept many notebooks full of my writing, which I would allow her to read. I remember her advising me to "do something with your writing" while I was in high school. I knew she was right, but it would take me many years before I would find the courage to show the world who I truly was.

✏️ Art Therapy Exercise

Draw a large house in the middle of a blank sheet of paper. Divide the house into the four sections that represent the areas in your life: relationships, work/education, personal growth/health and well-being, and leisure. Within each section, write down the types of activities and people you connect with or the kinds of things you can do to support your values in that area. For example, if you value humor, order, knowledge, and justice, write down under the work/education area the clubs, organizations, or jobs you are interested in joining or applying for, such as theatre, debate club, or a job focused on preserving human rights. If you find one area lacking, think about how you can make changes so your values are being expressed in that area of your life, and illustrate or write out your thoughts.

CHAPTER 12

Let's Talk about Goals

You've now identified areas of your life where you need to make changes. Setting goals will help you begin to improve your situation. Goals are actions that are guided by values. They are tangible. Goals will evolve over time, but values are a way of living, and they remain throughout a lifetime. This is why recognizing your values is vitally important to knowing what you ultimately want to achieve.

Goals keep your life going in the right direction. They are also good to have in place during times of stress or when that self-doubt monster comes lurking. During weaker moments, it's good to review your goals. They also keep us from returning to old habits that aren't good for us, for example, when we try to find happiness in a pint of ice cream or when we feel like skipping a few meals in an attempt to regain control over our life when everything else feels completely out of control. It's okay to have goals related to health and well-being, but when the *only* goals we have revolve around weight and our outward appearance, that's when a vicious cycle is created of trying to find happiness and self-acceptance by searching outside of ourselves as opposed to looking within to fulfill our purpose.

How do we set goals and take appropriate actions so we're living the life we're meant to live—according to our values? Refer to your value cards again and let's return to the topics of relationships, work/education, and leisure (let's leave out health and wellness for now; we will address it later). Decide which area needs your attention first, and set some short- and long-term goals. If you're struggling with this question, ask yourself which aspect of your life coincides the least with your values—that's a good place to start.

If you notice all three areas aren't working for you right now, don't stress. And don't attempt to tackle all of them at once. Choose one area to work on at a time. Use your journal to write down your goals to make them clearer and more attainable—you are more likely to succeed in acknowledging and achieving them when they are in writing. Below are five steps you can follow to formulate your goals.

Step 1: Summarize Your Values

I'm going to describe Step 1 as Dr. Russ Harris explains in his book *The Happiness Trap* (2008). Choose the area you are going to work on and write it at the top of the page. Next, write a brief description of how you will incorporate your values into that area of your life. For example, you've decided to formulate goals in the relationship area of your life, and you value honesty and world peace. Write: "In the area of relationships in my life, I value honesty and world peace."

Step 2: Set Long-Term Goals

What would you like to achieve over the next five years or within the next year? Long-terms goals can be anything you want them to be. Brainstorm ideas with your values in mind; try not to veer off of them. Your long-term goals should align with your values. Now, with your main destination in mind, use this long-term goal to inform your medium-range, short-term, and immediate goals.

Step 3: Set Medium-Range Goals

Look to the next few months ahead. What kind of goals can you set for yourself that will take you in your valued direction? If you are focusing on the area of education and work, medium-range goals are easy to determine because of time-specific academic calendars.

Step 4: Set Short-Term Goals

Short term goals are things you can do within the next few days and weeks that would be consistent with your values. Taking the example from Step 1, if you realize you don't have any relationships where you feel your world peace value is present, a short-term goal could be to find a group at school or in your community where like-minded people who share this value meet regularly. Attending a meeting like this could lead to the larger goal of cultivating the right relationships.

Step 5: Set an Immediate Goal

Finally, think about what you can do right now. If one of your values is for others to become more honest with you, one immediate goal that you can set into motion immediately is to be, in turn, more honest with your family and friends. Surround yourself with people who share this value or who would be interested in helping you obtain your long-term goal(s).

Let's visit our friend Stephanie again to illustrate how you can put all of this together. We last left Stephanie off at a college where she is unhappy. Her whole life is moving away from her values. What if, one afternoon, Stephanie decides to sit down at her dorm room desk and map out her life according to her values? She jots them down: creativity, ecology, achievement, compassion, fitness, fun, and God's will. These values will help her to set her goals.

Step 1: Stephanie Summarizes Her Values

Stephanie decides she needs to make a big change in her life regarding education and work. She wants to change her major to something that will fully support her values related to ecology, creativity, and compassion. Stephanie would summarize it like this:

In the domain of education/work, I value ecology, creativity, and compassion.

Stephanie isn't exactly sure yet how she will do this, but she continues to map out her goals.

Step 2: Stephanie's Long-Term Goals

Stephanie decides that in order to figure out what she really wants to do in five years and beyond, she needs to research careers. For now, she simply makes her long-term goals more broad-based according to her values. This is the beauty of using your values to determine goals—they help guide you in the early stages, when you're still unsure, until you come to solid conclusions. One of Stephanie's long-term goals, five years from now, is to study at a different university and graduate with a degree that aligns with her values.

Step 3: Stephanie's Medium-Range Goals

One of Stephanie's medium-range goals is to investigate new colleges and universities over the next few weeks and months in order to achieve her long-term goal.

Step 4: Stephanie's Short-Term Goals

Over the next few days, one of Stephanie's short-term goals is to visit the career center at her college to do some research and explore careers that are in line with her values.

Step 5: Stephanie's Immediate Goal

Stephanie's immediate goal is to call the career center and make an appointment with a counselor. Another immediate goal is to do some preliminary research online.

By simply making the appointment, doing online research, and writing down her goals, Stephanie starts to feel more positive. She finds herself looking forward to her appointment with the career counselor, and this motivates her to put on her workout clothes and go for a run. This good feeling stays with Stephanie, and she finds herself without her usual craving for a snack that typically gets her through her homework. This enables her to truly feel hungry when it is time for dinner.

As you can see, one small action step toward your values can trickle down and influence the rest of your life. The motivation to take care of yourself happens organically. The ability to feel true hunger returns, and eating for the purpose of nourishment and enjoyment comes back.

Health/Wellness Goals

Let's talk specifically about the health/wellness domain of your life. I'm going to suggest some very broad goals, which you can customize according to your own personal value system.

Step 1: Summarize Your Values

Write your values down and keep them in mind as you formulate your health and wellness goals. It's important for you to see your values in all of your goals.

Step 2: Set Long-Term Goals

Up until this point, you were probably setting long-term goals related to a specific number on the scale, a clothing size, or an ideal body type like the ones you see in the media or that belong to celebrities. These kinds of goals are good in that they are very tangible. However, for those who struggle with body image and eating disorders or disordered eating, this kind of long-term goal can be problematic. Instead, choose a long-term health and wellness goal that incorporates healthier habits and outlooks.

Pick one or two goals from each step (long-term, medium-range, short-term, and immediate). Record them in your journal.

- Accept and love my body
- Nurture my body with nutritious food and exercise
- Enjoy food and eating
- Experience the joy of not being at war with my body
- Minimize consuming highly processed foods and foods with high refined sugar content

Step 3: Set Medium-Range Goals
- Eat healthy and nutritious foods three times a day
- Plan to engage in some form of physical activity I enjoy several times a week
- Increase your nutrition awareness and knowledge

Step 4: Set Short-Term Goals
- Discontinue using food as a coping mechanism
- Find a physical activity I enjoy and can/will do regularly
- Do not deprive myself of food

Step 5: Set an Immediate Goal
- Only eat when I am hungry
- Be mindful of the sensation of being hungry (techniques explained in next chapter)

- Be mindful of the sensation of feeling full (techniques explained in next chapter)
- Eat mindfully (i.e., do not partake in any other activity while eating, and be aware of your senses of taste, smell, sight, and sound)
- Make sure I eat while sitting down in a peaceful atmosphere; avoid eating with people who fight with each other
- Throw away the scale; do not weigh myself
- Eat the foods I feel like eating
- Be aware of the moments when I eat when I'm not truly hungry
- Be mindful of my emotions before I eat

These are just a few goals that address your health and well-being from a broader perspective, with a sense of self-nurturing. See if you can brainstorm more goals for yourself. Notice that none of these goals are based on calorie counting or any type of "dieting" rules. By adopting this kind of attitude toward your body and food and by focusing on health and wellness goals in broader terms, you will begin to see how much more important the rest of your life is, and you'll find a better life balance. The purpose of these goal-directed exercises is to assist you in finding your passion and purpose. When you do so, you will feel empowered enough to make amends with your body and food; you will start living a life free from the emotional chains that were holding you hostage and creating unhappiness.

One last point regarding goal-setting: be certain that you are not setting yourself up for stress, anxiety, and ultimate failure as you formulate your goals. Your immediate and short-term goals need to be reasonable and attainable. Do not use goal setting to self-sabotage! I say this because I used to be the queen of setting unattainable goals for myself. And I'm going to freely admit to you that, once in a while, I still fall into some of my old habits. If I find myself spinning out of control because I've piled way too much on my plate, I step away from myself and make some adjustments. Because I'm aware of this tendency, I no longer beat myself up; instead, I laugh at myself for falling into old behaviors. Then I look at what's going on in my life that might be causing this: maybe I'm stressed or simply overly excited about a new project, and my dreams get in the way of realistic goal-setting.

In summary, be realistic with yourself as you set your goals. If the goal is not reasonable, make adjustments until it is more in line with your ability to achieve it in a set amount of time. To help you step away from yourself, read your goals as if a friend wrote them. What would you tell a friend? Treat yourself like you would treat your best friend.

My Story

When I first started grad school, one of my professors, who was an art therapist, gave us an assignment to create a piece of art that illustrated a life goal we were working on. She brought in magazine clippings, pipe cleaners, small pieces of fabric, rope, buttons, string, and just about any kind of crafty thing you could think of. We were also instructed to title our art. I entitled mine "Seeds of Change."

📝 Art Therapy Exercise

Use your creativity to illustrate your long-term goals with a collage or a piece of abstract art. Or create an artwork that illustrates how all your goals—from immediate to long-term—feel to you. For example, if you have a long-term goal of becoming a physical therapist, create an abstract illustrating your feelings of nurturing and excitement that come with the profession. Choose colors and shapes to depict those emotions or represent the school you'd like to attend to earn your degree. You could also use colors and shapes the represent the medical community or the American Physical Therapy Association of America.

CHAPTER 13

Listening to Your Body— Mindfulness and *You*

The topic of mindfulness is everywhere nowadays. Most of us are familiar with the basic principles of mindfulness, but there is also a sense of confusion. Some of us may think that mindfulness and meditation are the same, but they are not. Although practicing mindfulness is a form of meditation, being mindful is very different than meditating. Being mindful is about living in the moment; it is the opposite of multitasking. Practicing mindfulness means to focus on the here and now, aware of all your senses. Think about a dog when it is out on a walk—it is fully present in the experience. Anyone can engage in mindfulness right away, and it doesn't require training or a huge time commitment. You can practice being mindful while you're walking on the street, brushing your teeth, or doing chores.

Conversely, meditating needs to be learned and requires a certain amount of time and effort to train your brain to enter a meditative state. Both mindfulness and meditation are aspects of Buddhism. Mindfulness is just one of the many techniques utilized in transforming your thought process to reach a meditative state.

Mindfulness is becoming increasingly popular; as more and more studies are showing how it can benefit our health and well-being. The mind is a very powerful tool, and research reveals that learning how to become more mindful can change destructive thought processes (faulty thinking). Mindfulness is an excellent way for us to be healthier, happier, and less stressed in our daily lives.

How can mindfulness help eliminate food as a coping mechanism? In the earlier chapters, I discussed how important it is to pay attention to what you are eating and only eat without distractions. This is a form of mindfulness. Listening to your body and being mindful of your gut instincts and intuition is another form of mindfulness; it helps us understand our feelings better and what we actually want, so we don't have to turn to food. Lastly, all the art therapy projects throughout this book can be thought of mindfulness practices as well. Anytime you are fully present in the moment, such as soaking up every detail of what's going on and focusing all your senses on what's happening, can be called a practice in mindfulness.

Mindfulness can be utilized as a coping tool in life, specifically in managing thoughts and emotions. According to Dr. Russ Harris (*The Happiness Trap*, 2007, p.27), if we constantly run from our thoughts and feelings by distracting ourselves or hiding from the truth, we'll never find happiness or feel comfortable with who we are. Life will become more about avoiding the things that scare us, rather than true living. Dr. Harris has a term for this: experiential avoidance. Eventually, whatever we're trying to run away from will catch up to us one way or another. Dr. Harris goes on to explain how, when we run away, we will be unable to experience anything because we have spent all our senses and energy on avoiding. This is especially true when consuming food or restricting food is used as a substitute for facing pain and unpleasant feelings. If you are eating in order to bury thoughts and emotions, you will not be able to fully focus on enjoying your food. Conversely, if you are too focused on losing a few pounds and restricting your eating in order to gain control of your life, you'll be unable to process, accept, and handle the unpleasant or the uncomfortable. Avoiding thoughts and feelings means you're not fully present, which can lead you to become out of touch with reality. Another downfall of not accepting and addressing these root problems means they might trickle out into other areas of your life, creating even more issues instead of solutions.

For example, if you struggle with diets and gaining or losing weight, chances are the people around you have tried to help. And, quite possibly, some of them might have accidentally made things worse by creating a very uncomfortable atmosphere during mealtimes. Perhaps everyone around the dinner table is so focused on what you are putting in your mouth that it becomes impossible for you to enjoy your meal. Or perhaps your family and friends suddenly become the experts, commenting on everything you should and shouldn't be eating, which can be distressing. These kinds of experiences do not give us positive feelings. In fact, if enough of these negative experiences pile up on us, we'll begin to associate eating with being extremely uncomfortable. And if those thoughts and feelings, in turn, are not accepted and processed, they can become more painful and intense over time. This experiential avoidance then spreads into other areas of our life, and suddenly, we're declining going out for pizza with our friends after the movies or dreading food-filled holidays.

What are some ways we can practice mindfulness? Here is a list of practices that can help you to be more present in the moment, more aware of your body, and more in tune with your feelings and thoughts.

Mindfulness Practices

1. When you're doing mindless repetitive tasks, use that time in your day to simply focus on what you're doing and nothing else. For example, brushing your teeth in the morning can be a good time to practice mindfulness. Without any distractions, notice how the toothbrush feels against your teeth and gums. Pay close attention to the taste of the toothpaste and what it feels like as it foams up in your mouth. Being mindful is simply being fully present and noticing what happens to all your senses as you are performing an activity.

2. Take a walk without music. As you walk, notice your breath and how your feet feel on the pavement. Soak in your surroundings and look closely at the things you walk past. If you're in a very familiar space, try and find things you have not noticed before. For example, if there are trees along a familiar route, notice the detail of each tree.

3. Coloring is a good way to practice mindfulness and can alleviate anxiety. When you are coloring, focus on how the crayon, marker, or pencil feels on the paper as you move it. Reflect on the colors you choose and pay attention to how the color looks on the page. Notice the small differences between the darker and lighter shades.

4. Cleaning your room or doing the dishes is a good time to practice mindfulness. Think about what you are doing and spend that time truly focusing on your actions. Take note of the difference in your feelings before you begin the chore and after you finish.

5. As we've mentioned, eating at the table is another opportunity to practice mindfulness. Try to ensure that at least one meal a day is eaten with purpose and intent, without distractions. You'll find yourself enjoying the food more and feeling much more satisfied and nurtured.

These are just a few examples. Remember: you don't need formal exercises to practice mindfulness; mindfulness is really just about being super aware of your actions and connecting with all of your senses as you perform a task.

Lastly, when you practice mindfulness, you are connecting your mind and your body. Some of us have spent a considerable amount of time intentionally distancing ourselves from our body and ignoring the mind-body connection. As you attempt to repair this relationship, learn to be keenly aware of your body and what it is telling you. It takes time, but once you build this awareness within yourself, you will start to notice that life's challenging moments become a little easier to handle. Listening to your body enables you to be more in tune to your reactions to the world as life happens, whether you're standing at a crossroads or in a time of stress. Stress, especially, creates reactions in your body that can interfere with your ability to think clearly and continue down the right path. Conversely, an awareness of your body and mind will lessen the times when you wonder, "What was I thinking when I did *that*?"

My Story

I wasn't exposed to the concept of mindfulness until just a few years ago; however, when I look back on my daily morning runs during the weight-loss camp I attended as a teen, I realize I was already practicing mindfulness back then. At that time, technology wasn't as widespread or personalized as it is today, so plugging into an iPod or cell phone to listen to a music playlist while running wasn't an option. I still recall running over the same bridge every morning, which came up twenty minutes into the run. During the first week, by the time I reached the bridge I had to walk across it because I was so out of shape; my legs felt like two slabs of concrete. I barely made it back to the camp. After about four weeks into the seven-week camp, I was in good enough shape that by the time I reached the bridge, it actually felt good to be running. The only sounds I could hear were the inhales and exhales of my breath, my feet hitting the pavement, the birds singing, and the rustling of trees. I vividly recall the heat from the morning sun on my face and my shadow, which I watched as it "ran" in front of me. I wasn't aware at the time that those early morning runs had forced me to practice mindfulness!

Now, whenever I am at my lowest point or feel like I can't figure out my feelings or next steps to take in my life, I take a walk with the dog, without music, and focus on the present moment. I don't try and think about what I'm feeling or how to solve the dilemma on my mind. I just walk. I focus on my surroundings, my breath, my feet, my hands, and every other detail my senses are bringing in. Believe it or not, by the time I start to feel tired, my thoughts begin to make more sense, and I begin to come up with solutions. Sometimes, I figure out my problem before I even get home.

Art Therapy Exercise

Being fully present in the moment of creating art is a form of mindfulness. Repetitive actions or motions can help us focus fully on the moment or the task at hand, allowing us to be present with ourselves and our thoughts. Coloring is a popular form of creative mindfulness (which is why adult coloring books have become so popular).

Find something to color. Print out a coloring page from an online source or take a white sheet of paper and, with a black or blue marker, fill up the paper with intersecting circles, squares, or odd shapes with gaps in between them. Use crayons to color in the open spots. Notice the feeling of the crayon, marker, or pencil on the paper and how it glides across the page. Color with a light pressure, then apply more weight to create a darker hue. Use all of your senses while you color. What is happening on the page? How do your fingers and hands feel? What is the smell of the crayon?

CHAPTER 14

What to Do with the Pain in Your Life

Life is a challenge. Life is difficult. Life can be disappointing, frustrating, exhausting, and, at times, too much to handle. Sometimes life knocks you down to the ground with a punch so hard it feels you'll never find the strength to get up. If life hits you with a blow in the gut that is so forceful you can't catch your breath, it is time to ask adults for help or speak to a therapist.

This chapter focuses on the less traumatic challenges in life that still hurt us. This pain might come and go or remain with us like a dull toothache. Events can happen that make everything suddenly seem dark, lonely, and hopeless. Perhaps you are bullied by one person, and the next day twenty other students have jumped on the hate-train so that walking into school feels like wading in a sea of dread and despair. Perhaps you ran for president of a club and lost by only one vote. Or maybe a friend posts the most embarrassing, awful photo of you on social media, one that makes you look like a complete loser. These rough moments can feel overwhelming and bring about confusion and frustration if we're struggling with who we are or what we want in life.

In this chapter, we'll learn how to manage difficult times without turning to food. The idea is to put distance between the pain in your life and yourself, to seriously examine the difficult feelings that emerge, and to come to an understanding that these feelings are not permanent and will soon fade away.

To illustrate my point, let's visit Stephanie at her new college. Earlier, Stephanie realized she wasn't making decisions based on her values, so she went through the process of self-discovery and found a college better suited to her values and goals. Stephanie changed the way she thought about her life and found the courage to take constructive action by enrolling in a new college. She is now on the right path to live life on her own terms, instead of a life based on other people's values.

But what if about midway through the semester, Stephanie faces a challenge that is like a blast from the past. There is one class Stephanie worries about—chemistry. It is the one class she must pass in order to obtain her degree. In the past, Stephanie learned to face her negative feelings and overcame her anxieties surrounding chemistry. However, Stephanie's professor is giving her a hard time. She picks on Stephanie a lot and randomly calls on Stephanie, putting her on the spot. Stephanie is never able to answer her questions correctly. To make things worse, the TA (teaching assistant) whom Stephanie approaches for extra help makes her feel even more inadequate. Stephanie approaches her professor to propose doing extra credit work or retaking a quiz to raise her grade. The professor is rude, and she even challenged Stephanie's ability to finish college. Back in her dorm room, Stephanie finishes an entire bag of Doritos after crying her eyes out and talking to her friends. She and her roommate decide to go into town for French fries and milkshakes, and when they return to the dorms they proceed to eat dinner in the cafeteria. By the time they are back in their room, where they had planned to do some studying, they are both so uncomfortably full that they can't muster up the energy to do anything but watch Netflix.

If Stephanie does not deal with this situation in a constructive way, she will continue to have negative feelings and thoughts every time she steps into her chemistry class. She will suffer through the semester, constantly feeling inadequate, and probably eat her way through. If she continues to cope with the issue through food, her inadequate state of mind might affect her other grades as well. What's really unfortunate is that Stephanie doesn't have to feel this way about chemistry, the professor, or herself. She can change the way she thinks and feels about this whole situation. And I'll illustrate how.

Stephanie needs to accept her professor for who she is. This professor obviously has an issue with Stephanie that has nothing to do with Stephanie herself. I know this might not make much sense at first, but it is true. There are just some people you will encounter in your life who will conflict with you. This can happen for a number of reasons, and I will illustrate how to deal with difficult people in a later chapter. But, before we talk about actions, let's talk about how to deal with the thoughts and feelings in this scenario. First of all, Stephanie needs to listen carefully to her own thoughts while dealing with this professor. Some thoughts that pop into Stephanie's head could go along the lines of, *The professor is right. I'm stupid. I'm a loser. I'm not good enough; I'm not smart enough. Why am I even in college?*

Let's focus on the thought of "I'm stupid." We've already learned how to recognize destructive thoughts as "stinking thinking." If we accept, manage, and reframe this negative thought in the right way, we can change how we feel. When Stephanie hears "I'm stupid" in her head, she needs to first accept it. *Accepting* is not the same as *believing* (in other words, it is not true that Stephanie is "stupid"). Accepting is also not running away from the thought or avoiding it. Accepting means to allow that thought to be exactly what it is. *A thought.* Once she accepts the thought as a thought, she needs to step away from it. She can imagine the thought sitting on her shoulder, detached from her. Or she can imagine the thought as a balloon that is floating away from her. She can also imagine the thought as an annoying friend who insists on walking to classes with her and who won't leave her alone. Stephanie can waste time and energy hoping that this annoying friend will stop talking to her. Or she can continue to allow the annoying friend to walk with her, but also find other friends to accompany her as well, friends she can focus on. The same is true with our thoughts. Acknowledge them, allow them to be present, but don't let them be the focus of our life.

Once Stephanie has accepted the thought, her next step is to reframe or change the way she says the thought to herself. Instead of thinking, *I'm stupid*, Stephanie can think, *I'm having the thought that I'm stupid.* Suddenly, the thought loses its initial power, and Stephanie is able to recognize that she doesn't have to *become* her thought. She has taken a step back from the thought to view it from a new perspective. This new perspective opens Stephanie up to the possibility that the professor, the TA, and Stephanie herself simply don't think and communicate in similar ways. With this realization, her thoughts become less negative, her negative feelings begin to fade, and she can start to take appropriate action, such as finding a tutor who can explain concepts to her in ways she understands, finding a study group with students who are having similar issues with the class, or forming her own study group.

As you can see, this concept is different than simply trying to "think positively" or erase the negative thought. Imagine if we were to say to Stephanie, "Don't think that way. Just get that thought out of your head. Every time you think you're stupid, just think you're smart instead." Although this might work for a while, Stephanie hasn't given herself the opportunity to accept the thought as just a thought; instead, she spends a lot of energy pushing it away. Avoiding our feelings by hiding behind a pile of fries or devouring a pint of ice cream will only ease the pain for a short time (as we already know). We entertain a million thoughts a day. Some are extremely helpful, and some are not. We are human, so it is important to allow yourself to feel uncomfortable feelings and accept that they do indeed exist. Being human means having a bad day, not understanding something now and then, or not getting along with everyone we encounter over a lifetime. What's most important is to allow ourselves the space and time to recognize the thought for what it is: "I'm having a thought that I'm stupid, or I'm having the thought that nobody likes me at school." Then, step back from these thoughts and figure out what you can do to showcase your intelligence or become more connected to the people who care about you.

Now that we know how to manage negative thoughts and feelings that arise from situations outside of ourselves, let's talk about how to manage those that arise from within ourselves or that seemingly have no probable cause. To illustrate my point, let's go back to Stephanie. Stephanie has settled into her new college and things are going pretty well. However, she wakes up every morning with a feeling of sadness. She doesn't know why she feels this way—down, blue, crappy, or whatever word we use to describe sad feelings. When asked why she feels this way, Stephanie says, "I don't know." She also says, "If I were thin and beautiful, I would wake up every morning and feel great."

Let's tackle the first response, "I don't know." In order to help herself, Stephanie needs to spend some time examining the reasons why she doesn't know. This requires the courage to dig deep for an answer and accept it, an answer that will most likely create pain. My personal theory about painful feelings stems from one of my favorite pioneers in the field of psychology, Dr. Albert Ellis. Dr. Ellis argues that our true nature is to avoid pain. Imagine you're holding a hammer in one hand, with your other hand flat on a table. Would you be willing to take that hammer and smash your other hand? Absolutely not! It is the same idea with inflicting emotional pain on ourselves. However, as opposed to the hammer scenario, if we are brave enough to face and accept painful feelings, they eventually go away or become so dull we'll barely be aware that those feelings exist. Conversely, if we try to run from them, we are guaranteed to run toward other things that will increase our pain. Life will not get better. Stephanie's "I don't know" will eventually manifest into actions that will increase the likelihood of her increasing unhappiness.

Let's examine Stephanie's second response, "If I were thin and beautiful." Sure, feeling healthy and good about yourself can make you feel physically better. However, recall that being physically healthy and feeling good about your outward appearance comes from the inside. When we live according to our values and work toward goals that are vital to our existence, we'll feel at peace with ourselves. Confidence builds. Relationships prosper. We are purposeful and happy. These feelings manifest in how we carry ourselves, our facial expressions, and how we react to others. As a result, our outward appearance will improve naturally. Conversely, Stephanie's belief that happiness is tied to being thin and beautiful will result in her only working on her outward appearance, which will be futile. If Stephanie doesn't think past her appearance, she won't know what else to change in her life in order to find happiness within. This will leave her feeling unhappy, without knowing the reasons why.

To get to the bottom of Stephanie's despair, I'd ask her to tell me what thoughts are floating about in her mind whenever she's feeling depressed in the morning; I'd also raise other questions aimed at assisting her in uncovering the reason(s) behind her feelings of sadness and ineffective thoughts. Becoming aware of why certain feelings exist is the first step toward healing. Below are some questions you can ask yourself if you are in a similar situation as Stephanie. The intention behind this exercise is to isolate the thoughts that contribute to the pain.

Exercise

1. In your journal, write down a thought that seems to create feelings of sadness or suffering in your life.

2. How many times have you thought this way in the last week? (If you are unsure, simply write down a guess or estimate.)

3. What have you done to cope with this painful thought or feeling?

4. How effective has this been for you in the short term and long term?

5. When you think this thought and feel a resultant sadness, despair, or low self-esteem, what does your body look like? Are you slouching or hunched over; are your shoulders drooping?

6. Think about someone who could help you with the painful feeling(s). It could be a real person or an imaginary person. Choose someone who is wise and whom you look up to and admire. What would this wise person say to you? Write it down.

7. Think about the painful feelings again, and describe what you believe is the opposite of that pain.

Does the last question confuse you? According to number of experts, including Dr. Steven Hayes, who is known for bringing acceptance commitment therapy into practice, the opposite of someone's pain is what is truly meaningful to them in life. Feeling pain about something means you care enough to feel the pain. By identifying the opposite of your pain, you will discover what's important to you, what you really want, and what you need to do to get rid of it. This helps the pain feel a lot less . . . well . . . painful. For example, if your pain is caused by loneliness, the opposite of loneliness would be companionship or feeling part of a group. Or if your pain was related to feeling inferior, the opposite of that is confidence.

Now, keep this concept in mind as you read on. Once we discover what is important to us and what makes our lives mean-ingful, a whole new world opens up for good things to happen. Understanding your values, accepting life's challenges, and having the ability to be present in the moment as you travel through life are all positive ways of living. While you embark on this newfound road to becoming who you want to be, there is one thing that is almost guaranteed and bound to happen for you—and that's success.

Your Purpose/Meaning + Understanding Your Values + Accepting Life's Challenges + Having Present Moment Awareness = Success

Be true to yourself and think about what success means to you. Imagine for a minute how you would feel when you actually experience all the accomplishments that will lead you toward a life filled with purpose; imagine how successful you will feel in what you do every day. How great would that be? Bask in these positive feelings of success for a while, then take a step back and ask yourself: Do I have any fears surrounding the notion of success? A lot of times, we think, *If only I were successful, I would rule the world;* or *if only I were successful, I wouldn't feel so crappy about myself.* However, we rarely stop to think about the possibility of fearing success.

Have you ever thought that being successful might be scary? Another way of seeing this is to ask yourself if there have been times in your life when you had an opportunity to be successful, but you sabotaged yourself unintentionally to avoid the success. How much fear do you have when you think about a successful life? These might seem like silly questions. Why would I ask such a thing, and why on earth would someone not want to be successful? But this isn't about *wanting* success, it is about being brutally honest with yourself and knowing if you can be *comfortable* with allowing success to be a part of your life.

For some of us, life hasn't always been particularly easy. When life deals us a lot more criticism and shame instead of praise and rewards, success feels unnatural. These feelings are foreign, like being jolted out of familiar surroundings and transported to a foreign country while you are sleeping. You wake up somewhere strange and need to get acclimated to a new way of life.

If you've only ever been accustomed to hearing negative remarks and "put downs," it might feel really strange to suddenly hear compliments like "good job" or "well done!" If someone said, "We'd like to offer you a scholarship" or "You've earned a promotion" or "You've won an award," your first reaction might be, *What did you say? Me?*

Mull this over. How will *you* feel when success finally becomes part of your life? Feeling successful can be powerful, and the feeling of power can be foreign. Acquaint yourself with this possibility and be in tune with your inner world. While you travel down this new road and start to see things differently, know that it is okay to feel uncomfortable or awkward with success and a new sense of power. Disordered eating sometimes occurs as a result of feeling powerless, especially when the absolute *only* power you've ever possessed is related to your body, what you eat or do not eat, or whether you exercise or do not exercise.

My Story

There was a time in high school and at the beginning of college when I couldn't see myself for who I was; I was too caught up trying to be someone else. This "someone else" was wrapped in a perfect package, like the models and beautiful celebrities in the pages of magazines. I believed the key to happiness was grounded in being perfectly beautiful, which is what motivated and drove my eating disorder. Being occupied with food and dieting and my dream of having a perfect body distracted me from the real issue, which was feeling crappy about myself because of those false negative thoughts.

When I finally disconnected myself from my eating disorder, I discovered what I wanted in my life. I accepted and celebrated my strengths, as well as my challenges. However, I didn't realize I had one more missing piece of life's puzzle to figure out. I still didn't recognize the negative messages I played over and over in my head every day. Although I had already been exploring the idea of positive thinking, had taught myself to be confident in my looks and my body, and had let go of perfectionism, I was still unknowingly ignoring many negative thoughts that took up a lot of time and energy.

When I began to record my thoughts and feelings in a journal, I was able to recognize that I still thought others were better than me. My inner thoughts were based on the inaccurate thinking that other people were smarter, funnier, more creative, more successful, wealthier, and all around better than me. I had a classic inferiority complex that I was able to hide very well at times, and at other times it came through full force (and sometimes unexpectedly—yikes!). I had never addressed these thoughts before, because I didn't even know they existed. Writing these negative thoughts down and seeing them on paper in front of me was disturbing. Luckily, one other thing happened when I wrote those thoughts down—I could finally see how "off" and inaccurate they were. I also realized how much these negative thoughts were zapping me of energy. My feelings of inferiority and low self-worth not only created more sadness; they also drove my actions. At one point, I managed to stumble back on the right path, but after losing my sister to an addiction, I was pushed right back onto the wrong road. My guilt over her death consumed me, and I made decisions that turned out to be very destructive to my life. This guilt I felt stemmed, once again, from inaccurate thoughts. I thought I could have saved her from her addiction, which is not effective thinking. This ineffective thought pattern manifested in decisions that took me in the opposite direction I wanted to go. I was in the middle of the ocean, lost at sea, alone, and drifting, and it felt like I would never get back on the right path.

Eventually, I found the right therapist and learned all about Dr. Albert Ellis, cognitive behavioral therapy (recognizing negative thoughts and learning how to effectively manage them), and faulty thinking (inaccurate thinking). I learned to accept the sadness in my life without trying to ignore it or wrestle with it. I also did a lot of work to learn my life values and how to keep them in mind whenever I have to make a decision or a choice.

📝 Exercise 1

This first exercise might be a little challenging, but I have faith that you can do it. It will assist you in seeing and accepting that your thoughts are simply thoughts. As I've said several times, our thoughts do not have to define us or make us who we are. They are merely notions that arise out of our minds. Recall that inaccurate thinking can lead us to negative feelings, which can in turn cause us to take actions that don't align with our values and that are not in our best interests. This exercise focuses on ways you can distance yourself from inaccurate thoughts so they become less powerful and are reduced to exactly what they are: just words.

When we see our thoughts for what they are, the words lose power and we are able to either refrain from destructive actions or take actions that move us in the right direction.

1. I want you to think about a negative thought you often say to yourself. What is the worst thought you have about yourself? It might be something you've said to yourself in the past or something you hear inside your head daily. Write it down in your journal.
2. Now, I want you to condense that thought and those words down to one word—only one word. Write the word down.
3. Next, say the word out loud and rate the word on a scale from 1 to 100 on how powerful the word feels to you (1 being not powerful at all, and 100 being seriously powerful). In other words, when you say and hear the word, how do you feel?

4. Next, use the same 1 to 100 scale to label how believable the word seems to you. In other words, how true is it? Is this a fact? Is there proof that this word is accurate?

5. Finally, set a timer, and say the word as fast as you can, while still enunciating it clearly, for 20 to 45 seconds. You *must* stay within that time limit (Masuda et al. 2004). After doing this, answer the following questions.

   Does the word have the same amount of power to you?

   Does the word still feel as believable to you?

   Does the word feel as disturbing to you? Why or why not?

The purpose of this exercise is to experience the act of saying a word over and over again for a short period of time. This lessens the effectiveness of the word and its emotional impact. When a word is said out loud for long enough, it shows itself to be . . . just a word.

📝 Exercise 2

Look at the vision board you created (on page 93). If your vision board has changed somewhat since you've worked through this book, make those changes. Now, imagine that everything on the board comes true for you. Then, step back from the vision board and think about how you will feel when you are finally successful. How does having power in your life feel to you? Express this with some kind of art: on a big sheet of paper write out a list of words in bubble letters and color them or write them in different font types; or draw multiple pictures or one big picture that represents how you'll feel with power.

PART 3

Your Relationships with Others

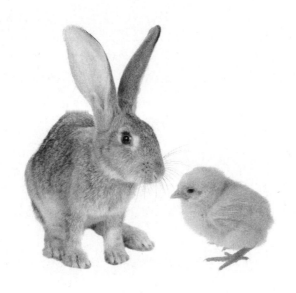

CHAPTER 15

Emotional Risk and Relationships

Knowing how to navigate your relationships is an important aspect of managing your life without using, or restricting, food. If you are to truly connect with people, you need to take emotional risks or be vulnerable. And being okay with vulnerability means being okay with unpredictability and accepting that nobody is perfect.

I've stated throughout this book that eating disorders or disordered eating are attempts to deal with life's challenges. Sometimes, eating disorders or disordered eating can snowball into something more serious; it can become such a large part of a person's life that food intake, physical exercise, and body image becomes the only focus in life. And most of the time, this happens as a result of faulty thinking, specifically black-and-white thinking or all-or-nothing thinking. Situations are either perfect or horrible. There's no in-between.

When we think about our relationships with others, black-and-white thinking doesn't work well because human relationships are not predictable. Sure, you can get a sense of someone, but we can't possibly know for certain what another person is thinking, and we can't expect anyone to be perfect. People mess up and accidentally say or do stupid things that can result in hurt feelings. Relationships are extremely complex, and an entire book could be devoted to how to manage them. In this book, I will simply explore a few main concepts regarding all relationships—with friends, family, lovers, work colleagues, etc.

All relationships require some form of vulnerability. Of course, your relationship with a teacher or a boss won't require you to be as vulnerable as committing to being someone's life partner. While vulnerability is a necessary component in human relationships, some people fear baring themselves in front of others, and they can easily avoid feelings of vulnerability by closing themselves off or hiding behind an eating disorder or disordered eating. Furthermore, for those who already suffer from eating disorders or disordered eating, destructive thoughts can reject, push out, and replace healthy ones so quickly you don't even notice them. Those destructive thought processes in turn seep into the relationships we have with others, creating even more distance between you and everyone else in your life.

To illustrate this point, let's use Stephanie again. When the family dinner table conversation revolves around how much she is eating or not eating or when they talk about her performance in school and in her other activities, the conversation transforms into an interrogation, and Stephanie eventually associates eating in a group with feelings of judgement, shame, and vulnerability. She grows to feel uncomfortable in any dining situation, fearing that she will be put on the spot by others, as though she is "on trial." Essentially, her past experiences create a negative emotional connection for her. However, if Stephanie is able to take a step back from those negative experiences and see them for what they are, past experiences, she will be able to dictate new experiences with new people and ultimately create new, positive feelings around eating with others. If Stephanie chooses instead to avoid dining with others at all costs, she will never have a chance to replace the bad memories with good ones. Avoiding social situations like this will negatively impact her social life. The first step for Stephanie is to recognize that she avoids these social interactions as a way to stop feeling vulnerable.

Feeling vulnerable is normal and healthy; it is necessary for deep human connection. The more intimate the relationship, the more vulnerable a person needs to be. People avoid being vulnerable in many ways, one of which is avoiding intimacy. In fact, many couples wind up in couple's counseling because one or both partners are unable to open themselves up to being truly vulnerable and intimate with each other. Romantic relationships evolve over time, and if one partner shuts himself or herself off from the other as soon as things get complicated (which they will), problems will arise.

Let's now create a scenario whereby Stephanie decides she is tired of struggling with social situations that revolve around food. She consults with a counselor at the college campus counseling center, and her counselor helps Stephanie review the situation in a new light. We've talked about the importance of accepting our feelings, which requires the ability to accept that a negative past experience had happened to us. We also talked about taking a step back from our thoughts so they don't define us.

Similarly, it makes no sense for Stephanie to resist the shame she felt at the dinner table every night or deny her anxiety when she told her parents that she got a C on her chemistry exam. What she *can* do is accept that this happened to her. This allows her to take a step back from those memories. The past does not define the present or the future. Nobody needs to keep living a certain way just because their past was crappy. People can choose to think, feel, and take actions in whatever direction they want to go. During the times when thinking about the past brings back strong negative feelings that trap us, you need to seek out a therapist or a professional who can guide you through the process of change.

In the 1930s, theologian Reinhold Niebuhr (1892–1971) wrote a serenity prayer that can help you think about the past. The prayer was published in a magazine in 1951 and popularized when Alcoholics Anonymous used a modified version in their meetings. Here it is:

> Grant me the serenity to accept the things I cannot change,
> the courage to change the things I can,
> and the wisdom to know the difference.

When Stephanie hears this prayer, she acknowledges that perhaps her past hasn't been so great but that she has the power to change her present and future. Stephanie begins to regret missing out on social situations she had previously avoided because she let her past dictate her present behavior. Stephanie decides she wants to change. She wants to take a risk and become more vulnerable. How can she do it?

A few girls Stephanie knows from one of her classes ask her to go for coffee. Stephanie says yes. She's a little nervous, and the upcoming date gives her anxiety. But Stephanie has interacted with these girls before, so she's fairly comfortable with the prospect of chatting over coffee (plus, it doesn't involve dining together). They meet and enjoy themselves. A few weeks later, Stephanie and the same group of girls decide to go to a movie and a dinner. Stephanie is nervous again, but she manages her anxiety because she really clicks with these girls; they have a lot in common, and they have all been very open and kind to her. The movie and dinner turn out great, and Stephanie realizes that not every dining situation has to feel like an interrogation.

Stephanie uses her newly learned coping skills to accept her anxiety and distance herself from past negative thoughts. She continues to hang out with the girls on weekends, doing all kinds of fun things. Stephanie also works on feeling more comfortable with opening up and allowing herself to be vulnerable. She accomplishes this by being completely honest with herself and the three of them. She understands that being honest means allowing her friends to see every aspect of who she is, and she relates with them in a genuine way. For example, she says no if she is not interested in a particular activity. She also allows them to see her true self— when they open up and share intimate details about themselves and their past, she does the same without judgment.

One night, her friends ask her to go out to dinner with a group of people Stephanie doesn't know. Stephanie understands this will require her to be even more vulnerable. She agrees, but a few days later her anxiety gets the best of her. She tries hard to diffuse her apprehension by distancing herself from her thoughts, but every day she keeps thinking about how difficult this will be. She will have to sit down and have a meal without knowing everyone at the table. There will be four other girls and boys, and there will be many unknowns. Stephanie isn't sure that she can deal with the situation.

There are two ways Stephanie can deal with her anxiety. First, she can recall her past and accept those nightly family dinners that were filled with shame. She can also accept that her parents love her and were doing what they thought was best for Stephanie; they were most likely raised by their parents in the same manner. This thought is an act of forgiveness, which frees up Stephanie's emotional energy to move forward. This also allows Stephanie to accept those events as past difficult moments that can no longer hurt her. She can look on those memories for what they are: memories.

Second, Stephanie can decide to focus her energy on the present. She can allow her old memories to fade into the background and focus instead on fully connecting with her friends, whether old or new. She can choose to be fully present in the moment of the dinner and not waste her energies on the past or her old relationship with food.

Finally, if Stephanie values friendships, she can remind herself that this new way of thinking will put her on the right path toward what she values in life. Stephanie's commitment to her choice of action is in line with her values, which gives her the strength to follow through—she knows it's the right thing to do. And no matter how it turns out, at the end of the evening Stephanie will have had an experience that proves she is capable of allowing herself to be vulnerable.

During the dinner, Stephanie allows her anxiety to be present—but only as an annoying party guest seated at the table next to her, and she doesn't waste any energy trying to push it away. Once in a while, her anxiety friend laughs too loudly and interrupts her focus on the conversation, but she simply re-focuses herself back to what is important to her. The evening is fun and filled with laughter. Stephanie's experience proves to her that it is indeed possible to share a meal with complete strangers who accept and embrace her for who she is and who are living their lives according to similar values.

A note of caution: know that vulnerability does not mean allowing others to step past boundaries you are not comfortable with. Being vulnerable means trusting yourself and your gut instincts. Be vulnerable according to your life values. Opening up to others should create an exchange of mutual respect, which means others should respect your boundaries and differences, if you respect theirs, too.

My Story

In my novel *Wish I Could Have Said Goodbye*, the main character, Carmella, struggles with vulnerability throughout the whole story. She meets a boy, Howie, shortly after she loses her older sister to an accidental drug overdose. While dealing with the pain of her loss and grief, Howie walks into her life, and Carmella has to act. She is challenged with either allowing herself to be vulnerable or passing up the opportunity to get to know this new guy. I can't give away the ending, but I can tell you that Carmella learns a lot about vulnerability throughout the book.

Writing fiction does require storytelling skills, but it also requires truth from the author. There was a time in my life when I felt very much like Carmella, especially in high school. In fact, I spent most of my life being very guarded, and I did not allow myself to be vulnerable. It became easy for me to remain this way because I could hide behind my eating disorder. Eating disorders are a very easy way to avoid dealing with emotions. By obsessing over my body, dieting, and exercise, I didn't have time to be vulnerable. In my friendships, I sought out the types of people who weren't interested in being vulnerable with me. You'll know when you're in the company of people who refuse to be vulnerable because you never truly *know* them. These friends don't talk about their feelings, their pain, or their hopes and dreams. They don't share intimate details about themselves and are not interested in talking to you when you need to discuss real issues. They don't want to know how much something in your past or present hurts you or what you think about when you see something beautiful. These friends usually don't talk about anything other than which Kardashian is getting divorced or which one is seeing a therapist for compulsive shopping. They usually enjoy gossiping about others but rarely (if ever) talk about their own feelings. They don't talk about pain, and they don't open up and reveal their true selves to you.

Eventually, as I worked on myself and my issues, I started to grow emotionally. I found friends I could sit with and talk to for hours over coffee and whom I got to know better and better. They accepted me and all my crap. They are friends I still have today. Being vulnerable can be scary and complicated. But as long as you know yourself and who you are, you will be able to trust your instincts. Most important, listen to your gut.

📝 Art Therapy Exercise

Find any type of small- to medium-size jar with a lid. If you don't have one lying around the house, hobby and craft stores or dollar stores will sell them. You will also need red colored paper, markers, scissors, clear tape, some magazines, and a glue stick.

The purpose of this exercise is to illustrate how to protect yourself while allowing yourself to be vulnerable with others. As much as vulnerability is vital to relationships, at the same time it is important to recognize the times to exercise self-protection.

Create a paper heart cut out of red paper. This will represent you and the emotional well-being you need to protect. Place this red heart inside the jar. Next, think of ways you can protect yourself from emotional danger. Examples of self-protection can be affirmations, positive quotes from other people, good thoughts that can push out negative ones or "faulty thinking," etc. You can cut out images of people in magazines to represent friends or family whom you can turn to for support and who will help you feel stronger and more stable. You can draw, write, or cut out images of activities that help you feel more secure or assist you with sorting out your thoughts. While you're thinking about this, don't leave out the cases in which we hurt ourselves. We often hurt ourselves by allowing destructive thought processes to rule our life or push out the constructive thoughts we have.

Once you have gathered all those ways in which you can protect yourself, tape them onto the outside of the jar or put them inside, next to your heart.

CHAPTER 16

Assertiveness

Being assertive means behaving confidently, expressing to others what you think and believe in a direct way. The concept of assertiveness is easy to understand. However, putting these traits into actions can be difficult, especially if adults or authority figures have made you feel ashamed for who you are. And when food becomes the only way of coping with life, learning to say no assertively, politely, and with respect can be a challenge.

It is very important to understand the difference between assertiveness and being aggressive. Being too aggressive is just as destructive to relationships as being incapable of asserting oneself. Being assertive does not make the other person feel shame. Assertiveness is simply standing up for who you are, what you want, and what is right, while also respecting the other person in the process. On the other hand, you can think about various reality television shows that showcase good examples of highly aggressive people. If you want to see a good example of aggressiveness in comparison to assertiveness, just watch an episode of *Dance Moms*, a reality television show about a group of teen and tween competition dancers in the Abby Lee Dance Company—and their moms. The mothers on the show attend every rehearsal, and they all travel together to competitions. Whenever the owner of the dance studio, Abby, and the moms get into a disagreement, which is very often, they deal with one other in an aggressive manner. They are disrespectful toward one another, scream and yell and use abusive language, and sometimes even use physical force. Nia's mom, Holly, is one of the rare moms who acts assertively without being aggressive—she says no when she needs to, and even when she is in a highly emotional state, she remains calm, chooses her words carefully, and does not attack, shame, or blame the other person.

How can we be assertive in difficult situations? The easy way out could be to turn to food to manage the problem; or we can choose the more uncomfortable but long-term solution of confronting someone using assertive rather than aggressive behavior.

Let's visit Stephanie again to illustrate how to effectively handle a conflict or difficult situation using assertive behavior. At her new college, Stephanie enjoys her classes, the club she has joined, and the friends she has made. She gets along extremely well with her roommate, Maria, except for one thing—Maria is a night owl. She studies all night and stays up until two or three in the morning. Fortunately, she doesn't have classes until noon, so she can sleep in. Stephanie, on the other hand, is a morning person. She likes to get up early. Her first class is at eight a.m., she is done studying by ten o'clock in the evening, and she is ready to go to sleep around eleven. Stephanie values education and her health, but she is losing sleep when Maria stays up with the desk light on; she hears the tapping of her computer keys or the music seeping out from her ear buds. Although Maria tries to be quiet, Stephanie is awakened by the noise, especially when Maria gets up to go to the bathroom at two in the morning. Stephanie needs to talk to Maria to see if they can work this out.

If Stephanie were to return to her old methods of dealing with problems, she might attempt to eat her way out of the bad situation. We know this would result in her feeling bad about herself and frustrated that her situation is not getting better; she might even begin gaining weight, and her grades could suffer. You can see how being assertive and facing this challenge is very important for Stephanie not to fall back into old habits.

Stephanie has grown and changed over the past few years. She does think about eating her way out of her problem, but quickly realizes that a hundred chocolate milkshakes will not change anything. Instead, she sets out to handle this difficult challenge in a healthy way. She understands that she doesn't know her roommate too well yet and is unsure of how she will react. Stephanie also knows that imagining or projecting the outcome of a conversation will not be helpful, as it is impossible to predict how any other person will react in conflict, especially one she's not known for very long. Stephanie works hard to avoid getting caught up in inaccurate thoughts about the outcome. She focuses on what she can control, which are her words, thoughts, feelings, and actions. She knows she needs to remain calm and clear and express herself with sincerity and without shame or blame toward Maria. Being assertive requires you to remember your values, while understanding and believing you deserve to get what you want. Being assertive doesn't mean getting what you want or need at the expense of someone else. Being assertive means feeling confident that, together, they can figure out a solution that will benefit both of them.

Stephanie begins the conversation with a positive statement. She lets Maria know she values their friendship, but she is losing sleep, which is affecting her grades. One of the tricks to keeping communication lines open and to lessen conflict is by using *I* statements in place of *You* statements. *You* statements attack and blame, while *I* statements do not threaten or shame the other person. Instead, *I* statements honestly communicate what you're feeling. For example, saying, "I run away from conflict so it's hard for me to talk about this" opens up the communication. This statement makes it more likely the other person will hear what you're saying. Here is another good *I* statement: "I respect your body clock and the fact that you're a night person, but I'm much more of a morning person." The statement is not phrased as an attack. Stephanie tries these methods, and she also lets her roommate know that staying up on weekends when there's not class the next day is not a problem. Stephanie adds honestly, "It's difficult if I can't sleep on weeknights because I'll get worried and stressed about my grades." Stephanie is vulnerable with her roommate and lets her know her true feelings. Finally, she asks the question, "How can we figure out a solution so you can stay up late to study and I can get my sleep?" This statement requests a solution to the problem that works for both parties.

Being assertive always includes a request. Asking for a solution from the other person is important. You're not simply telling the other person how you feel. Be honest and open about your feelings first, then make a request if you want change to happen. Being assertive is like a math equation: *I feel [insert feeling] + when an action or event happens + I'd feel better if something else happened or something changed + Can we make a change? (request) = Assertiveness*. In Stephanie's case, it would look like this: "I feel stressed out when I can't sleep because of the noise or light in the room. I'd feel less stressed and worried about my grades if I could sleep better. How could we figure out a way for you to study late and for me to get better sleep?"

There are many solutions. Maria could go into the lounge to study. Maybe she'll try getting computer work done earlier in the evening and save all her reading for later so she's not making any noise. Maybe Stephanie decides to use ear plugs and a sleeping mask.

This is just one example of being assertive to solve a problem. If you feel you need help in this area, seek out an assertiveness training class or a therapist who can assist you. Becoming more assertive takes patience and practice, especially if you've experienced a lot of shaming in your life or have only experienced negative experiences when you've attempted to speak up for yourself. And don't forget what I said earlier: negative memories and thoughts are simply images in your mind, and new, constructive ones can take their place. You just have to step out of your comfort zone and take a chance on change!

My Story

When I struggled with my eating disorder as an adolescent, I was an expert at keeping everything I thought and felt bottled up inside of me. I didn't know how to express myself. When conflict happened, I had no idea how to deal with it. Conversely, when I was much younger, in grade and middle school, I was very comfortable being assertive. My best friend made it even easier for me because she was as sensitive and honest as I was. Conflicts between us never felt like conflicts because we were straightforward and respectful to each other. I could be honest with her about what I wanted, and she would return the sentiment. We always discussed our options about what we wanted to do. We made a pact in first grade: if one of us didn't want to do something, we would not do it. Or we would split our time doing the things each of us wanted to do. It was easy to be assertive with each other because we were so much alike.

But then I got older and met new friends, and things became much more complicated. I assumed everyone was as straightforward and sensitive as my best friend. I didn't know that other people held back, weren't honest, and played "head games," which I just wasn't ready for. When I came across these complications, I was lost. What I didn't understand was the amount of stress I put on myself to be perfect and how I demanded that the rest of the world be perfect, too. I didn't realize that people might hurt me accidentally and that if a friend hurt my feelings once, that didn't necessarily mean they hated me. I wasn't aware of the possibility that they might have screwed up, could have been having a hard time with something else, or were simply in a bad mood. When I did speak up and express myself, I assumed that meant our friendship was over.

Eventually, I met some really great friends in college who taught me how to be assertive among others. We were honest with each other, which allowed me to feel comfortable being assertive with them. Sometimes I did stupid things when I tried to stand up for myself, and sometimes I didn't express myself in the most effective way. They could have shunned me for my hurtful words and actions, but they understood I was simply trying to figure out how to navigate life. They forgave me, and I learned how to forgive myself. I finally accepted that perfection is not possible, and I stopped putting pressure on myself to be perfect.

✏️ Art Therapy Exercise

If you feel you'd like to express yourself more assertively, draw a doormat in the center of a white piece of paper. Next, write all the benign phrases you often say to others instead of expressing how you truly think and feel, for example, "Whatever you want" or "I don't mind." Then, write phrases on the doormat that express how you feel about yourself, including words that represent how you feel when your needs are not being met.

Turn the paper over. Draw a stick figure and a word or thought bubble coming out of its mouth. Inside the bubble, jot down all the ways you can express yourself assertively to others. If you recall times in your past where you missed an opportunity to be assertive, write down what you would have said if you had been more comfortable asserting yourself in that moment.

CHAPTER 17

How to Deal with Difficult People

You know who they are. They are the people you avoid at school, work, or in your family. They are the people who can't seem to find anything positive anywhere. They are unpredictable and impossible to please. Maybe you've had a boss like this, a friend, a coworker, or a relative. The most important thing to remember is that they are difficult for reasons you will probably never understand. They could be reacting to personal issues that have nothing to do with you. An encounter with a difficult person can impact your mood in a negative way or feel so toxic that you want to run far away from them, but make a mental note that they are possibly unaware of themselves and how their behaviors impact others; they could even be suffering from their own private pain or trauma.

All this is easy to say when you're not in the heat of the moment. Dealing with a difficult person takes patience, and it is extremely important that you try to avoid judging them. Running away from difficult people or pushing aside negative feelings toward them, especially if you use unhealthy coping mechanisms, is not an effective solution. Deciding to handle a difficult boss by listening to him or her rant and rave at you for no good reason and then burying your feelings in a tub of ice cream when you get home after work is not effective or healthy. Instead, see the situation for what it is and recall that you have control over how you think and feel, but you cannot control others. Their anger or difficulty is about them, not about you.

Note that the situation changes if you encounter a person you feel physically threatened by or who is violating any kind of boundary. If your gut tells you to flee the situation, heed the warning. If a person makes you feel unsafe, consult an authority figure, an adult, or a friend immediately. For example, a coworker who is touching you inappropriately is not simply a "difficult person"; they need to be reported.

Here are a few ways to manage a difficult person whom you can't avoid. First, take a really deep breath and let it out. If you want to take a few deep breaths, go for it. As you exhale, imagine that you are letting out all the stress created by this person. Next, think about what's going on with your body. Do you feel anger bubbling up? Take more deep breaths and remain calm. Remind yourself that only you are in control of your feelings.

Secondly, be aware of how people like this attempt to control others with their difficult behavior. Is the person manipulating you? Do they act nice to you initially, but then turn around and talk about you behind your back? Are they constantly nasty to you? Do they never make eye contact with you? Are they distant? Difficult people are usually self-absorbed, and their words and actions tend to be all about them. If you can't figure out how a difficult person comes to a certain conclusion, it's a sign that their words are all about them, so don't discount your first reaction. If you are confused by any accusation or conflict, you can always take some time before you respond. Finally, remember to never take their words and actions personally.

Lastly, don't engage with difficult people. This doesn't mean you need to be a doormat. Difficult people tend not to accept anyone else's point of view, and they're not interested in hearing opinions besides their own. Simply allow the other person to say what they need to say, then take some time to respond. Sometimes, these people are simply looking for someone to argue with, and in this case it's not worth your time to engage in a senseless fight. Respond to difficult people with neutral statements. You can say things like, "That sounds like it was a difficult situation for you" or "I'm sorry to hear that." Being assertive, and not aggressive, with difficult people is another great method to solve conflict. If you feel trapped with this person, find a way to walk away from him or her. If this is a boss, coworker, or someone on your dormitory floor, limit communications with him or her as much as possible.

Lastly, if you are stuck with having to deal with a difficult person for an extended period of time, try to find compassion within yourself to understand where they are coming from. Attempt to see if they are responding to a personal pain or problem in life, and try to understand that their actions and words are likely a result of them trying to gain control over their hurt.

Ideally, spending as little time as possible with difficult people is the best scenario. Being around toxic people can zap you of your time and energy. Difficult people are usually stuck in ineffective and faulty thinking patterns, which might seep into your thinking. If you recognize this starting to happen, find ways to avoid spending time with them.

Here is a list of ten tips that summarize how to deal with difficult people:

1. Be assertive, not aggressive, with them. Avoid being angry. This will get you nowhere.

2. Be aware of the other person's level of anger, so you can be in control of your own emotions and keep them in check.
3. Be neutral. Don't be a doormat, but don't argue. Respond with neutral words.
4. Be accepting of them, while remaining at a distance.
5. Be polite and respectful, without being phony. Keep time with them short.
6. Be aware of what kinds of issues set them off and avoid hitting their "hot buttons."
7. Be patient and compassionate without letting go of your values and what's good for you.
8. Be a good listener. Focus on both their needs and your needs, not arbitrary actions or issues.
9. Be aware of your own boundaries and issues.
10. Be safe. Listen to your gut. Difficult people are not abusive or immoral. Know the difference.

My Story

Difficult people are even more challenging to deal with when you already feel bad about yourself. When I was at weight-loss camp, I encountered a camper who was an extremely difficult person to be around, especially when we were all learning more effective ways of coping with life and working hard at changing our negative thinking and attitudes into more positive ones.

To be honest, this girl was not manipulative or trying to cause trouble with anyone. She was simply very difficult to get along with because she was very unhappy and struggling to come to terms with a lot in her life that we were all too young to understand. There were about five of us in this little group. She would get on everyone's nerves by talking about her boyfriend 24-7, whom she would be away from for seven weeks. At first, we were all sympathetic. Every day, we would listen to her talk about her broken heart at breakfast, lunch, and dinner. During our nightly runs after dinner, she talked about it, too. She would phone him from the camp phone every night after our run (we didn't have cell phones back then). Then she would come back to the dorm and talk about how much her heart was breaking and complain about her life.

After a few weeks of this, we all began to lose our interest and patience. We didn't talk to our camp counselors because we didn't know it was going to get worse. The four of us would try to change the topic of conversation to cheer her up. We didn't realize it, but we were working harder at trying to mend her broken heart than she was. I'm not proud to admit this, but eventually we all began to avoid her. We felt guilty for our actions, but we were unable to handle someone so determined to remain stuck. Our motivation to avoid her became stronger as the days went on. Eventually, she realized what was happening and felt even more hurt—her new camp friends were rejecting her. Although we apologized, we weren't very sincere. After the camp counselors intervened, we tried to include her again, but she was so hurt she ended up staying in her room all day and all night, refusing to participate in anything. A few days later, she left camp. Looking back, we could have dealt with her more effectively using some of the strategies I mention in this chapter. We could have consulted with adults at the camp, and we could have changed our behaviors. It is difficult to know what would have happened if we had done things differently.

I have come across numerous difficult people in my life, and the strategies I've mentioned in this chapter work best for me. Sometimes, people will just get under your skin, and in the heat of the moment all logic can go out the window. This is why it's always best to check yourself and your feelings first before you respond. Managing your thoughts and feelings, which you can control, is the best strategy for dealing with people in general, especially the difficult ones.

✏️ Art Therapy Exercise

Fold a sheet of paper in half, either vertically or horizontally. Flatten the paper out; the fold is a dividing line. On one side of the paper, draw what it feels like to be with people who are easy to get along with. On the other side, draw what it feels like to be with difficult people. They can be abstract and metaphorical drawings.

PART 4
Putting It All Together

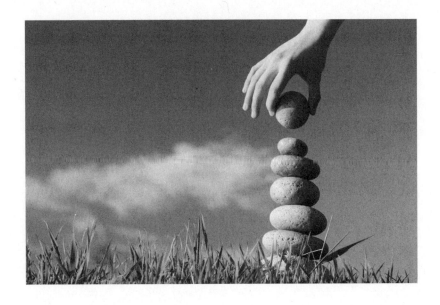

CHAPTER 18

What Is Your *Why?*

Asking yourself this simple question will give you strong insight into who you are and what you want. Knowing why you do what you do and why you think what you think gives you the power and freedom to make choices based on what is best for you. If you live life by this premise, you will not need to depend on food to cope or restrict food intake to gain control. During difficult times, especially if you feel you might fall back on old beliefs and destructive habits, ask yourself "What is my *why?*"

Knowing your *why* is about knowing what gives your life purpose and meaning. Asking and answering this question often will help you discover what motivates you and what makes you happy. Why do you get out of bed every morning? Why do you love to go to concerts? Etc. It is important to discover your life meaning and how it is related to your values and goals. When life gets challenging and painful events happen, holding on to your meaning will remind you of what's really important.

Just as Dr. Albert Ellis discovered how humans naturally tend to be negative and think in ways that can feed into our vulnerabilities, Dr. Viktor E. Frankl argued that some people who live through tragedies don't just survive after their trauma; they thrive. He wondered how some people are able to withstand challenges far better than others, and he set out on a quest to identify these differences.

Dr. Frankl was a renowned neurologist, psychiatrist, and survivor of the Holocaust. He discovered early in his career (before the Holocaust) that if people are connected to meaning in their life, they are able to overcome tragedies and live a happier, more content life. He argued that human nature is motivated by purpose in his most successful book, *Man's Search for Meaning* (1946). I've summarized the basics of his philosophy and theory on how you can live a meaningful life here.

1. Life always has meaning. Even in the most miserable situations, and even if we don't understand the "why" during our darkest moments, meaning exists. Eventually, we will have an answer.
2. The primary motivation for living is to find meaning in life.
3. Every person has the freedom within themselves to discover meaning in what they do and what they experience, or at the very least, in the stand they take when faced with a situation of unchangeable suffering.
4. A human being is made up of body, mind, and spirit.
5. It's important to listen to your spirit. It is your guide in life.
6. Regardless of what we go through in life, we always want to know the question *why*.
7. Don't be distracted by things that hold you down or hold you back.
8. Pay close attention to your ability, creativity, ideas, potential, and spirit.

Discovering meaning in your life is about knowing exactly who you are and what you want to become, and knowing your values and goals in turn is a good start to defining this meaning. You have the power to make your own choices according to your values, and these choices will put you on life's right path.

Another way to discover your personal meaning is knowing what you can offer the world through your own unique character, creativity, and relationships. When you share a piece of yourself with others, you give yourself a chance to live with meaning and discover what is most meaningful to you. Fully accepting yourself and your past is also a way of getting to know who you are.

Finally, situations arise in our life that require us to respond. Sometimes it's easy to forget that we have the power to choose and control our attitudes. Even if we don't have a choice in what happens to us, we always have a choice in how we respond and what kind of attitude we take. If we look at our responsibilities as opportunities to discover meaning in our life, we'll get closer to what's important.

My Story

As you know, one of my passions is playing the guitar. I learned almost all the Beatles' songs and played their songs every day until my twenties. I became such a huge fan of the group, particularly John Lennon, as he was both a great musician and a huge advocate for peace. I admired everything he did to make the world a better place. John Lennon's "why" was clear to the entire world (as was Yoko Ono's). At the time, I wasn't fully aware of my own values, passions, and life purpose, but I knew I believed in the same things John and Yoko did; I wanted to someday make the world a better place.

It was an exciting time for all their fans when the album *Double Fantasy* came out. It felt like a constant celebration of two people who were admired for their music and also for what they stood for and represented—they were determined to spread peace in the world. John Lennon used his art to bridge gaps between people. Although he was world famous, he was known for always taking the time to sign autographs and connect with his fans. As most of us know, this trust in humanity was how he was killed outside his home in New York on December 8, 1980, when I was a junior in high school. I was shocked and devastated. I attended the worldwide memorial, standing with thousands of people in the middle of Grant Park in Chicago, singing "Give Peace a Chance" together.

I can still remember the moment like it was yesterday. I even remember the black pants, sweater, and coat I wore. Although my "why" was not as clear to me then as it became later in life, it resonated with John Lennon's. I believe in the power of peace, love, and positivity. Everything I do, think, and feel is always about trying to do what's best for others and humanity, while being true to myself. I don't dare to compare myself with John Lennon, nor am I even remotely close to his level of talent, abilities, vision, and greatness, but the values he represents has been a part of my life since I was ten years old.

The choices I've made throughout my life have taken me down many roads. There was a time in my life when I consistently made decisions that put me on a path to nowhere. I went backwards and in circles, never moving forward. This was around the time I experienced the tragedy of losing my sister.

There were times when I felt completely lost. I collapsed emotionally, unable to take one more step, but then the nagging continued inside of me, and I felt I could not rest until I got back on the right path. I never gave up hope, and I never stopped moving. I didn't know it then, but what had motivated me to press on was the greater search for my "why."

Sometimes life can feel like too much to handle. There are times you should take a break. Rest and regroup. Take care of yourself, build yourself up, and then think about your "why."

✐ Art Therapy Exercise

For the final exercise in this book, go back to your list of values. In your journal, write down a value and answer the question: Why is this value important to you?

Look at all your answers and try and find a common theme. Summarize and write out this theme in a sentence or two. This will help you to answer the simple, yet profound, question, "What is your *why?*"

One Last Thought . . .

I hope the words and exercises in this book have assisted you in finding a new way to cope with life's challenges. I also hope that, through my story, you are able to see that you're not alone in your struggles with body image, food, disordered eating or eating disorders, or life in general. I also hope you will keep the image of the two roads going in opposite directions in the forefront of your mind, especially when things get complicated or you feel overwhelmed and lost.

I'd also like to congratulate you for taking a step toward a better life. Learning who you are and what you want can be a challenge, especially if you're used to only pleasing others. Simply recognizing that something has to change is the first step to get on the right path. Step two is deciding to take some kind of action to improve your life, and step three is actually taking the action. Working through the process of self-discovery and finding new ways of coping means you're on your way to a healthier and more fulfilling life.

You made a choice when you decided to read this book. That choice will empower you to change, and it will lead you further and further down the right road. No matter where you are in terms of your journey, know that life is a process of decisions and choices. Loving yourself for who you are will give you strength when times are tough. And during the most challenging moments, go into your toolbox and find the right tool to help you cope. I hope you practice using the tools you learned about in this book. Continue to expand your toolbox and discover more tools along your journey.

We all need to keep learning and growing, especially when it comes to ourselves and our mental health. We live in time when we're bombarded by an endless stream of information, and the world seems to be in so much pain and suffering. So now, more than ever, it is important to take care of ourselves and the people we care about. Make it a priority to connect with yourself every day. Remember to practice mindfulness, and remember to practice gratitude and forgiveness. And most important, remember that loving yourself and others is the most powerful thing we can do as humans.

About the Author

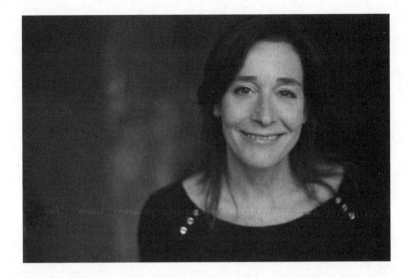

Shari Brady is an award-winning author who loves to write about life's biggest challenges and heartaches. Her debut young adult novel, *Wish I Could Have Said Goodbye*, won numerous awards within the first six months of its release. In addition to writing books, she's also a licensed professional counselor. When Shari's not working as a therapist, writing, or immersed in a new creative project, you'll find her hanging out with friends, walking the dog, or laughing hysterically while binge-watching sitcom reruns on Netflix with her two teenage kids. Shari is a native Chicagoan who lives in the northern suburbs with her son, daughter, and their shelter dog, Betty Queen Elizabeth. You can read more about her and her books at www.sharibrady.com.

Where to Go for More Information

These professional organizations listed below are resources if you want more in-depth information on eating disorders and disordered eating. This is not a complete list.

Academy for Eating Disorders: aedweb.org
Eating Disorders Anonymous: eatingdisordersanonymous.org
Eating Disorder Referral and Information Center: edreferral.com
National Association of Anorexia Nervosa and Associated
    Disorders: anad.org
National Eating Disorders Association: nationaleatingdisorders.
    org
Bulimia dot com is a useful resource for eating disorders and
    body image: bulimia.com

For More Information on Health and Nutrition
Center for Science in the Public Interest (CSPI)
To subscribe to the Nutrition Action Health Newsletter
go to www.cspinet.org
Center for Science in the Public Interest
1220 L St. N.W.
Suite 300
Washington, D.C. 20005

References

Abramson, E. 2001. *Emotional Eating*. San Francisco, CA: John Wiley & Sons, 2001.

Follette, V. M., and A. Vijay "Mindfulness for trauma and post-traumatic stress disorder." In *Clinical handbook of mindfulness*, edited by F. Didonna, 299–317. New York: Springer Science + Business Media, 2009.

Follette, V., K. M. Palm, and A. N. Pearson. 2006. Mindfulness and trauma: implications for treatment. *Journal of Rational-Emotive & Cognitive-Behavior Therapy* 24, Issue 1, pp. 45–61.

Gladding, S.T. 2016. *The Creative Arts in Counseling* (5th Ed). Alexandria, VA: American Counseling Association.

Jackson, J. L. and R. C. Hawkins. *Stress related overeating among college students: Development of a Mood Eating Scale* (unpublished manuscript, 1980). Copywrite Linda J. Jackson and Raymond Hawkins II, 1980.

Chapter 3

American Psychiatric Association: Diagnostic and Statistical Manual of Mental Disorders (5th Ed.). Arlington, VA: American Psychiatric Association, 2013.

EAT-26 Self Test, retrieved from http://www.eat-26.com.

Chapter 5

Clark, D. A., A. T. Beck, and B. A. Alford. 1999. *Scientific Foundations of Cognitive Theory and Therapy Of Depression.* New York: John Wiley & Sons.

Burns, D. 1999. *The Feeling Good Handbook.* New York: Penguin Group.

Damasio, A. 2000. *The Feeling of What Happens.* Boston: Mariner.

Ellis, A. 2001. *Overcoming Destructive Beliefs, Feelings, and Behaviors.* Amherst, MA: Prometheus Books.

Ellis, Albert, and Robert A. Harper. 1975. *A Guide To Rational Living.* Chatsworth, CA: Wilshire Book Company.

Freeman, A., J. Pretzer, B. Fleming, and K. M. Simon. 2004. *Clinical Applications of Cognitive Therapy* (2nd ed.). New York: Springer.

Harris, R. 2008. *The Happiness Trap.* Boulder, CO: Trumpeter Books.

Webb, J. 2014. *Running on Empty.* New York: Morgan James Publishing.

Chapter 7

Hoek, H. W., and D. van Hoeken. 2003. Review of the prevalence and incidence of eating disorders. *International Journal of Eating Disorders*, 34, no. 4, 383–396, http://www.anad.org/get-information/about-eating-disorders/eating-disorders-statistics/.

Chapter 8

Ten Steps to Positive Body Image adapted from:
https://www.nationaleatingdisorders.org/learn/general-information/ten-steps.

Chapter 10

Miller, R. M. and S. Rollnick. *Motivational Interviewing*. New York: Guilford Press.

Chapter 12

Harris, R. 2008. *The Happiness Trap*. Boulder, CO: Trumpeter Books.

Chapter 13

Harris, R. 2008. *The Happiness Trap*. Boulder, CO: Trumpeter Books.

Chapter 14

Hayes, S. 2005. *Get Out of Your Mind & Into Your Life*. Oakland, CA: New Harbinger Publications.

Chapter 16

Burns, D. D. 1993. *Ten Days to Self-Esteem*. New York: HarperCollins.

Chapter 18

Frankl, V. 1959. *Man's Search for Meaning*. Boston: Beacon Press.